The Spiritual
Heart

Meditations for Health and Happiness

The Spiritual
Heart

Meditations for Health and Happiness

Bruno Cortis, M.D.

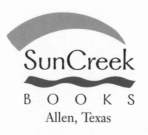

SunCreek

B O O K S

Allen, Texas

Send all inquiries to:
SunCreek Books
An RCL Company
200 East Bethany Drive
Allen, Texas 75002-3804

Telephone: 800-264-0368 / 972-390-6300

Fax: 800-688-8356 / 972-390-6560

E-mail: cservice@rcl-enterprises.com

Website: www.ThomasMore.com

Printed in the United States of America

Library of Congress Catalog Number: 2002109631

5702   ISBN 1-932057-02-1

1 2 3 4 5   07 06 05 04 03

I dedicate this book to you, my dear reader.
The healing of the physical heart
lies primarily in your spiritual heart.

ACKNOWLEDGMENTS

The spark for *The Spiritual Heart* was ignited in my heart six years ago. Many people have nourished the flame:

My parents and Aunt Amelia,
with their immense dedication, generosity, and love.

My brother Nello and my sister Leda,
who have left a great void in my heart.

Dr. Carleton Whitehead, my teacher of spirituality.

Dr. Deepak Chopra, a mystic leader and supportive friend.

Doctors Bernie Siegel, Jerry Jampolsky, Herbert Benson,
Joan Borysenko, Larry Dossey, Dean Ornish, Gary Zukav,
Paul Pearsall, Michael Mercer, Thich Nhat Hann, and
Claire Sylvia, who have inspired me with their works.

Theresa di Geronimo and Kathryn Lance for editing the
book proposal and the outline.

Debra Hampton and Thomas More Publishing
for valuing the manuscript and giving it life.

John Sprague for helping me
to communicate clearly my feelings.

My wife Pia and my children Veronica and Maximillian,
for their constant support and great love.

And finally my patients, who gave me the privilege to see
into their hearts and appreciate their wisdom and humanity.

CONTENTS

INTRODUCTION

From the Heart of a Cardiologist

Within our body lie two domains: the domain of the mind and the domain of the heart. If you are like most people, you are much more attuned to your mind than you are to your heart. In fact, you probably seldom think about your heart, unless you feel it pounding from running for a bus or you are unlucky enough to develop heart disease.

The mind, on the other hand, constantly demands our attention. It is, after all, primarily a reactive system, driven by the unsatisfied need of the ego for power and control. Our mind is materialistic. It seeks independence and it's judgmental and impatient. It is like a dictator, constantly demanding and commanding.

The heart, in contrast, is driven more by spiritual concerns, by love. Our heart seeks connectedness, self-expression, and fulfillment of our deepest needs in life. Our mind thinks, but our heart feels. Our mind is materialistic; our heart is spiritual. It is to help you become aware of the spiritual nature of your heart that I have written this book. My purpose is to help you understand how, if you take care of your heart and listen to it, it will take care of you. The result will be not only a reduction in your chances of heart disease, but an increased awareness of your deeper purposes in life.

You may wonder how an awareness of your spiritual heart can help your health. The truth is that health by definition is a state of complete physical, mental, and spiritual equilibrium. Although we used to believe that the mind and body are two separate entities, we now know that all facets of our being are interconnected. Everything that happens to our bodies and our minds affects the heart on some level. Every thought we have, every feeling and emotion we experience affects the heart. I'm sure you know from experience that just thinking of something exciting or frightening can change your heartbeat.

THE SCIENTIFIC BASIS
FOR THE SPIRITUAL HEART

Do not be misled by the word "spiritual" in the title of this book. Some will think that the issue here is of a spiritual nature only and, as such, not grounded in reality or physical science. I feel that it is important right at the beginning to provide scientific information that validates and gives substance to the concept of "spiritual heart."

We all know that the heart muscle is nourished with oxygen and nutrients by the coronary arteries. As we grow older, some of us are predisposed to the deposition of cholesterol within the arterial walls. Our heart is governed by two branches of the autonomic nervous system, the sympathetic and the vagal. The first accelerates the heart function, while the second slows it down.

In the morning hours, our body's physiology, the so-called circadian rhythm, changes. An increase in the sympathetic tone causes a rise in heart rate, blood pressure, oxygen consumption, and stress hormone levels. The coronary arteries undergo vaso-constriction with a decrease in lumen size and reduction of the blood supply to the heart (ischemia). In addition, the platelets become sticky and the blood has an increased susceptibility to form clots. All these changes predispose the occurrence of a heart attack, especially during morning hours. So it is of critical importance to prevent this cascade of events by reducing the sympathetic hyperactivity and achieving balance in the autonomic nervous system.

Balance is proper not just to the physical domain, but also to the spiritual. Since the element of stress contributes so much toward trig-gering all these negative changes, it is critical that we modulate our emotions and, in essence, our spiritual life.

THE MOMENT OF TRUTH

I first became interested in the spiritual aspects of the heart through my experiences as a cardiologist. Strangely, it was at a low point in my life, a moment when my work no longer felt fulfilling. At that time, my life seemed to be dedicated to waiting at the hospital for the next cardiac victim. I was tired of seeing young people die of heart attacks. I was tired of seeing the faces of spouses and children whose loved ones never came home from the emergency room. I was tired of seeing chests split open for surgery, or learning that someone else had been brought in dead on arrival. I was tired of dealing with the human body as a collection of parts disconnected from the essence of the person.

In short, I had come to realize that what people needed was to not get sick in the first place. My interest had shifted from disease to health—from patients to people and my objective evolved into becoming a teacher of health, and, specifically, someone who teaches people how to take care of their heart.

Sadly, in our society, people usually learn this lesson from disease, if they are lucky enough to survive. In the case of heart attacks, the lesson is sometimes too late, because one person out of three does not survive. The current statistic for heart attack deaths in the United States is 1,400 a day. The total number of deaths each day in the U.S. because of cardiovascular disease is 2,600.

It's a little like the plague—almost a million people a year die of cardiovascular disease—but we are so accustomed to it that even the media ignores it. In the past, it was thought that heart disease was for men only. Now we have discovered that women also develop heart disease—in fact, 250,000 women die of it every year. Heart disease has become the number one cause of death in men as in women. It is an equal opportunity killer.

For these reasons, I created a conference room in my office for my patients and their families. We would meet periodically, show slides on how to control risk factors such as hypertension, high cholesterol, diabetes, stress, and smoking. For a while, I even called a psychologist and a dietician to give classes. The patients wanted even more. I began to speak of the pain I felt as a physician when somebody in the hospital was not doing well; I shared my tears with families when somebody died.

When I opened my heart, a miracle happened: The patients began to share of themselves, not the same way they talk to the physicians in the examining room—they manifested themselves as persons. Their smiles and their happiness became my smile and my happiness. We hugged each other; we discovered the incredible beauty of being supportive. As we conducted these conversations, my interest in the spirituality of the heart increased and I began to examine the content of my own heart. I was accustomed to praying, or meditating, but looking into the content of my heart was really very revealing.

What a joy it is to just close your eyes and let your heart talk. Most of the time, we relate to each other by asking questions and expressing thoughts, opinions, and judgments. Judgments rule our lives. How different it is when you let the voice of your heart be heard. It is then that you have the clear ability to communicate. It is a communion of feelings and emotions. You discover your values. You discover there, within your heart the strength to make decisions that can change your life.

It was my heart that told me that the values I cherished were not respected in the land where I was born. It was my heart that told me to move to the States and begin a new life. When I left my parents, my friends, my brothers and sisters, everything I had accomplished in thirty years, to start a new life here, it was my heart telling me, "Go. Create the life that you want. Be the person you would like to become. Find new people to love."

I discovered that one of my greatest joys was that of self-expression. I began to ask people, "Do you ever talk to your heart?" Many just said no; they prayed instead. But, some said yes. Some of my patients had learned on their own to communicate with their spiritual heart. I remember Mary, a middle-aged woman who had been to the emergency room numerous times with an irregular heartbeat. One day, she decided to talk to her heart. "I don't want to go to the hospital any more," she told her heart. "I don't want to be stuck in a room and have to pay all those hospital bills. I don't want to be away from my family and I don't want this to keep happening."

Suddenly, her heartbeat became regular again. Mary discovered for herself that just by communicating with her heart, she solved the problem. On the way to the hospital she felt the difference. What a phenomenal experience! I began to tell people this story. I encouraged them to communicate with their heart, express their gratitude.

ONE DAY, I opened the Bible in search of the words that could express my mission. It was a coincidence but the words I read were, "Take care of the heartbroken." This is what I mean to do with my life. In 1995 I wrote a book called *Heart and Soul.* In that book I wrote a chapter on the spiritual heart, "Your Faith and Your Heart." That one chapter has taken my life in a new direction that now becomes the core of this book.

We all need peace, love, and a meaningful life. This book shows a pathway to fulfill this dream and the way is through your spiritual heart, living in your heart. In this book you will learn meditation, how to use your heart intelligence, how to communicate with your heart, and how to see through the eyes of your heart. You will know inspiring heart patients, but, most of all, you will discover yourself and your spiritual nature. Being in touch with your spiritual heart will raise the level of your consciousness, and this will bring you closer to God. Ultimately, this experience will change your life and allow you a new freedom.

CHAPTER ONE

Mind, Body, Spirit

We are not sent into this world to do anything
into which we cannot put our hearts.
—JOHN RISKIN

SPIRITUAL MEDICINE

If you look at the early history of medicine, where medicine and spirituality coincide, priests were the doctors because every disease was considered supernatural in origin. Only those who had the power to deal with the spirits had the ability to heal. Hypocrates (370 B.C.) described this as the healing power of nature. We have a physician within and we can heal ourselves.

When Greek and Roman physicians began to ask for money to pay for medical attention, a separation between medicine and spirituality began to develop. Finally, with the scientific revolution and all the major advances in the medical profession—the development of antibiotics, better anesthesia, progress in surgical techniques—the separation was complete.

However, we all desire some form of spiritual consolation. We seek an inner space where we can find peace and rest, a place where our faith resides, a solid ground that is independent from the changing world around us. We have come full circle. We are now demanding the return of spirituality. Now, more than ever, people are recognizing the need for the spiritual component to their lives and their health.

PERSONAL EMPOWERMENT

My education focused on identifying the disease and taking care of it. All the rest was irrelevant. But when I began the cardiac support group in my office, I realized that there is more to medicine than diagnoses and treatment. I discovered the full humanity of my patients. They began to hug me, to cry, to open their heart, to express their deepest feelings. They showed no reluctance in describing their experiences, even those of a spiritual nature. I became convinced that spirituality is essential to medicine.

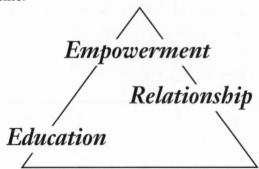

When individuals maximize their relationship with their physician, the end result is patient empowerment through a collaborative effort toward a common goal: the patient's well-being.

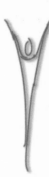

In addition to being the source of your physical strength, your heart is endowed with the spiritual qualities of love and wisdom. You can use your spiritual heart to gain control of your life. But to do this you must listen to your heart, connect with your heart, and take responsibility for your heart on both the physical and spiritual level.

Now I was working with each patient in a partnership, informing, educating, and empowering the patient. The final result was that I began to teach them meditation and to practice with them on a regular basis.

This path led me to further my own personal and spiritual development. The realization came to me that, in addition to being a muscle, the heart is endowed with divine qualities: love, wisdom, and a tremendous source of power.

I shared these principles with my patients and they rejoiced that they had this spiritual fountain within themselves, this inner light, this vital force.

THE HEALTHY HEART

The heart is a powerful muscle that beats over a hundred thousand times a day and pumps two thousand gallons of blood. Though we sometimes sense that it is filled with many different feelings, it is hollow inside. The four chambers of the heart fill with blood and then pump it one way out. The right side takes in partially oxygenated blood in the receiving chamber *(atrium)* and

17

pumps it from the second chamber *(ventricle)* to the lungs, where it releases carbon dioxide and becomes freshly oxygenated. The blood then travels to the *atrium* on the left side of the heart, where it is pumped via the left ventricle to the rest of the body. The primary route for sending out fresh blood is the body's main artery, the *aorta*. From the aorta, the blood enters the arteries that branch out from it as if it were a tree. Each branch has branches in descending sizes, going down to the twigs on the ends which are capillaries, tiny arteries with thin elastic walls that can open or close as the body's needs dictate.

The heart also has a blood supply of its own; the two main coronary arteries and their small branches that surround the heart like a crown *(corona)*. How does the heart function? Well, by providing the whole body with oxygenated blood and nutrients.

THE MODERN EPIDEMIC

The most common heart disease is arteriosclerosis, hardening of the arteries, which is due to the deposition of cholesterol within the wall of the artery and with the progressive narrowing of the lumen. There are two types of arteriosclerotic blocks that we call plaque. The first is characterized by a small amount of cholesterol and the covering of this plaque is thick. It is like the roof on a house. This is called a fibrous cap. We define this type as stable plaque because it has less tendency to break.

The second variety contains a large amount of cholesterol, the fibrous cap is thin, and it is more susceptible to rupture. This we call unstable plaque. When the fibrous cap ruptures, a sequence of events leads to the formation of a blood clot. And then a heart attack.

In recent years, the key realization that has emerged is that the majority of heart attacks occur in persons who have arteries that have become narrowed less than 50 percent. This comes as a surprise because we always thought that it was the arteries with 90 percent blockage or more that were the culprits.

Why does this occur? It happens because, as we said, the heart attack is caused by plaque that ruptures. It is the vulnerability of the plaque, not the narrowness of the coronary artery, that causes the problem.

Another element that may contribute to a heart attack is what we call a coronary spasm. In other words, the lumen of the artery, the inside diameter, constricts because the muscle fibers in the wall of the artery contract. The key point is the following, and it is a paradox: we have a heart attack caused by an artery that is less than 50 percent narrowed because of vulnerable plaque. We do not know why the plaque ruptures, or why it ruptures mostly in the morning, or why frequently on Monday mornings. It has been postulated that the hyperactivity of the sympathetic system is the primary cause of the changes that predispose one to a heart attack (these are described in the introduction). What an ideal ground, then, to reduce the sympathetic tone with meditation, prayer, or spiritual intervention!

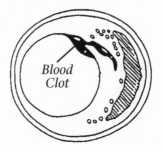

Cross section of an artery showing partial blockage and vulnerable plaque.

Blood Clot

There is another important statistic: the majority of people who die following a heart attack die of an arrhythmia, an irregular heartbeat (ventricular tachycardia or fibrillation). Only 20 percent of the victims have a heart attack. This emphasizes the importance of keeping the heartbeat regular, and the regularity is also related to a balance of the sympathetic and the parasympathetic systems. The overstimulation of the sympathetic system could increase the likelihood of arrhythmias. Focusing on the spiritual reality helps create a psychological and spiritual balance that is essential to our well-being.

HEART FACTS FOR MEN AND WOMEN

Women suffer heart attacks and heart disease just like men. Here are the facts, as provided by the American Heart Association, 2002.

As previously cited, 2,600 individuals die each day in the United States from cardiovascular disease—an average of one death every thirty-three seconds. This represents about 60 percent of the total deaths in the U.S. In 1999, 445,871 males died of cardiovascular causes (46.5 percent), compared to 512,904 female deaths (53.5 percent). Other major causes of death recorded for 1999 were cancer (549,838), accidents 97,860, and AIDS (14,802), with breast cancer deaths totaling 41,144 and lung cancer deaths at 62,703. The tobacco industry targets women by exploiting the association of having a slender figure and smoking.

Although the above statistics don't bear it up—one in thirty female deaths in 1999 was from breast cancer but one in 2.4 was from cardiovascular disease—most women are more afraid of breast cancer than they are of cardiovascular disease. The statistics are frightening. Two hundred fifty thousand people die suddenly each year of coronary heart disease without being hospitalized (usually from cardiac arrest due to ventricular fibrillation). The total cardiovascular deaths each year for people fifteen to thirty-four rose from 2,719 in 1989 to 3,000 in 1996. And the death rate increased by 30 percent in young women, especially African American women.

Doctor Marianne J. Legato, M.D., author of *The Female Heart* (Quill, 2000), describes the categories of women at risk like this: (1) the Type A woman—who hides her anger and frustration and learns to smile; (2) the nice girl who can't say no because she wants to be liked and admired—she tries to do ten times more than possible, like staying up all night making cookies or trying to run the church fundraiser; (3) the doormat—she has a subordinate, passive nature but hides a lot of hostility (you might find her in a high-performance job with low pay); (4) the neglected caregiver—she makes sure everyone in the family gets a checkup, for example, but forgets herself; (5) the woman on overload—she's continually under stress because she's handling two or three jobs at a time, working at home, at the office, and who knows where; (6) the isolated woman—one in five women will lose their husband between the ages of fifty-five and sixty-four; the resulting social isolation promotes illness.

What's a woman to do? Doctor Legato advises women to not be on call twenty-four hours a day, but to find a place where they can rest, identify what makes them happy, begin a sport activity, exercise regularly, and spend at least an hour a day just for themselves. Women, obviously, juggle multiple roles—as homemakers, as wage earners, as family caretakers, mothers, and wives. They are the ones who experience the conflicts when a child is sick or injured and they are at work. Women tend to have many more necessary activities than men—shopping, preparing meals, cleaning, and childcare—and of the total workload some work is paid and some is not, although the unpaid work is very important. Their activities tend to be more frequent, yet less flexible.

Wives report feeling responsible, even for their husbands. Unwinding at the end of the day is more difficult for them. A study performed on the blood pressure and stress level of both genders reports that after 5:00 P.M. the blood pressure and hormone levels of men drop, while they remained elevated in women. Also, the work stress in women's coping strategy may increase because of tendencies toward more weight, less physical activity, more anger, more smoking. And while men have cut down smoking by 20 percent, women have cut down by only six percent. One in three women of child-bearing age is still a smoker. The average age of a first heart attack in men is 65.8 and in women it's 70.4. The coronary heart disease rates after menopause are two to three times greater than prior to menopause. Myocardial infarctions without pain, so called silent heart attacks, are statistically more common in women than men: 35 percent to 28 percent. According to the Framingham Heart Study, 50 percent of men and 60 percent of women who die suddenly of coronary disease have no previous symptoms of this disease.

The major risk for women after menopause is a change in their lipid values, with an increase in LDL (low density lipoproteins), also called bad cholesterol because it forms deposits in the arterial walls, and a lowering of the HDL (high density lipoproteins), named good cholesterol because it keeps the arteries free of plaque. Smoking is also dangerous because it lowers the HDL and increases the risk of death 30 percent. Women who suffer from coronary heart disease experience different symptoms than men. They have more shortness of breath and nausea, and more atypical symptoms such as back pain and jaw pain—they have less chest pain and sweating.

Females are usually affected at an older age, but they tend to have more comorbidities such as diabetes, hypertension, and obesity. The diagnosis tends to be made late. And there is less intervention and less rehabilitation. In terms of diagnosing coronary heart disease in women, the treadmill gives false-positive results about 50 percent of the time, so physicians rely more on stress-echo and thallium tests.

In a recent article in the *Review of Cardiovascular Medicine* (2001, number 4, p. 181), authors Jane Leopold and Alice Jacobs affirm that women who suffer acute coronary syndrome, which means unstable angina or acute myocardial infarction, and who present themselves for interventional procedures, generally have characteristics that put them at higher risk specifically, they are older and they have a higher incidence of hypertension, diabetes, and congestive heart failure. Plus, there are technical problems that increase the complications of interventional procedures because of the smaller diameter of their coronary blood vessels.

In *Hurst's The Heart: Manual of Cardiology* (McGraw Hill Professional Publishing, 2001), Robert O'Rourke, et. al., observe that women more frequently describe symptoms of angina with emotional and mental stress, they tend to arrive at medical care longer after the symptoms have begun than men, they have received less thrombolitic treatment, aspirin, or beta-blockers, and fewer women receive interventions in the way of cardiac catheterization, coronary angioplasty, and bypass operations. And a final observation is that women experience a higher percentage of lethal first-time myocardial infarctions.

A common denominator of paramount importance for men and women who suffer from heart disease is their family. The heart problem becomes a family problem and everyone in the family is affected. It is like an emotional earthquake in the life of many persons. So think of the daily consequences: the total number of heart-related deaths each day is 2,600; this represents twenty-six hundred families deeply affect by this tragic event, and for a lifetime.

USING YOUR HEART TO GAIN CONTROL OF YOUR LIFE

How can we use our heart to take better control of our lives? We can be in touch with our hearts. We can use our "heart intelligence." We can grow in awareness that our heart gives us signals of comfort or discomfort according to circumstances. If we attune ourselves to these signals we can guide our lives toward healthy behaviors. When our body talks to us it is up to us to listen and try to understand the message.

This is especially true with the heart. Remember that the heart bears the load of our physical as well as our mental and emotional activity. Stress can affect the heart as it does any other body system. It may tell you "I am in trouble." "I am feeling overstressed." "I am not getting enough oxygen."

Just what are these messages? Perhaps the most common warning of impending heart trouble is called *angina*. Angina consists of chest pains which are the result of a reduced blood supply to the heart commonly brought on by physical activity or emotional stress. Angina is not always experienced as pain in the chest. Sometimes it feels like pressure or tightness in the chest, neck, arms, jaws, or upper back. Often if is accompanied by palpitation or shortness of breath.

One patient described her angina as "a cramp in my chest going completely to the back." Another patient said it was "like a big weight on my chest." Some patients, especially diabetics, may have no pain and experience dyspnea or fatigue that is disproportionate to the degree of effort they are making.

Arrythmias or irregular heartbeats can also be a sign of trouble. The most common arrhythmia is called the skipped heartbeat. (It is actually a premature contraction.) It feels like a palpitation or fluttering in the chest, and can be harmless.

Other arrythmias can cause the heart to beat too fast, or too slow. If these conditions persist they can lead to a variety of symptoms—lightheadedness, fatigue, loss of consciousness, even death. Arrythmias can be provoked by high or low levels of certain electrolytes in the blood, by use of cigarettes or drugs, or by a reduced blood supply to the heart (ischemia).

Emotional stress can also bring on arrythmias. While an occasional skipped beat may be nothing to worry about, continuing or recurrent arrythmias are important messages from our body and should be checked out. Sometimes your heart gives you little warnings that it is trouble. Angina and even heart attacks can be painless. It is estimated that 35 percent of the population, most of them middle-aged men, suffer from silent ischemia, which is associated with electrocardiographic abnormalities, but no chest pain. According to Eugene Braunwald (*Heart Disease*, W.B. Saunders, 2001), episodes of silent ischemia have been estimated to be present in approximately half of the patients with angina.

In essence, in order to rely on your heart to be in control of your life, you must become responsible for your heart. Trust in your doctor is not enough. Having all the tests in the world are not enough, especially if you don't know what the results are and how you must act on them. Medical tests and procedures have saved many lives but the real solution lies with you taking responsibility for your own health. This responsibility may involve changing your diet, stopping smoking, learning to control your inner life. It will be worth it, I promise you. It is important that you, as a patient, maintain an active role and be willing to work with a physician wholeheartedly.

BEING IN TOUCH WITH YOUR HEART

Consider this fact: The heart pumps 2,000 gallons of blood per day and beats 100,000 times each day, which adds up to nearly a million heartbeats every ten days. This merits the heart receiving your attention.

Usually, the heart symptoms are considered like an alarm and prompt us to take action, such as calling a friend, taking a medication, or rushing to the emergency room. Why wait until you're in trouble to connect with your heart. Wouldn't it be more reasonable to start communicating with your heart now, while you're well? The following exercise will show you how.

Exercise

When I place my right hand over the left side of my chest, I become aware of my heartbeat; in a few moments the sensation becomes less forceful. It's as if my heart knows that I'm in touch with it. The change in tempo and strength that I feel with my hand tells me that somehow the heart longs for touch—and by touch, I mean love. Try this yourself. Put your right hand over the left side of your chest and feel your heart, feel what happens to your heartbeat.

Start to communicate with your heart—you will notice that your heart talks back. Within your heart is an infinite intelligence that is sensitive to your needs. So pose a question to your heart—ask your heart for help. Right now I'm asking my heart whether or not I will continue to generate enough ideas for this book, and my heart is answering: "Continue to work on yourself, and have faith. The answers will come as you need them."

Once you begin your heart talks, there will never be an end to them, because your heart rejoices in communicating with you. Your heart loves intimacy and attention. The more you become aware of the spirit, the more you discover how much it does for you. I suggest that you continue these heart talks every day. You will notice the changes in your life. With an increased awareness as a spiritual being, you transcend the self-imposed limitations of the material world.

LISTEN TO YOUR HEART

Isolation is one of the most difficult aspects of battling illness. I think constantly about my patients who are tethered to heart-monitoring equipment and day after day lie alone staring at the ceiling of the coronary unit. To help these people stave off the inevitable fear, anxiety, loneliness, and depression, I decided to record a series of audiocassette tapes for inspiration and to remind them that they are not alone. I call these tapes my "Spiritual Heart" tapes. They are designed to provide emotional and spiritual tools for healing. I would like to share one of these messages.

NOTE: You may wish simply to read and reflect upon the following meditation, or you may want to read it aloud into a tape recorder and play it back while you sit quietly and listen with your eyes closed.

Meditation

We all have a spiritual heart
and this heart is never sick.
It is a perfect heart, a divine heart.
It is a heart that will live forever.
When we leave this planet,
our heart will continue to live.
It is this spiritual heart that I am describing now.
Please listen to your heart.
Listen to your deepest needs,
to your dreams,
to your goals.

Listen to your own heart.
It is unique and eternal.
"Do not let your heart be hardened,"
    says the Bible.
Be attuned to your spiritual heart,
    which is your perfect companion.
It can be your guide in the difficult walk of life.
It can be your light.
It can become an angel leading you
    to the spirit of God within.

Listen to your heart.
    Do not move away.
Stay close to your heart.
No one loves you more than your own heart.
It is a love that is silent, gentle, kind, and forever.
I believe that if you attune yourself
    to your spiritual heart
    you will never be sick at heart.
Your spiritual heart has a healing power,
    which is beyond your understanding.
It is a source of the greatest energy, creativity, and love.
Show your heart gratitude
    and take good care of it.

Feed it with spiritual thoughts,
    with moments of friendship,
    with moments of thanksgiving
    for being the source of your life.
You may never feel lonely again.

In talking to your heart and living in your heart,
you discover a fortress of safety, an island of peace,
a center in your spiritual universe.
Heart-to-heart communication is the deepest
and most meaningful form of contact.

Do not close your heart to others.
Do not be afraid to love.
The love you give will always come back to you multiplied.
The language of the heart is universal.
Speak that language.
Let your heart reach out and be reached.
Sense the unity of your heart with others,
the fundamental sameness within our individuality.
The child that you were lives in your heart.
Talk to your inner child;
encourage, help, and hug him/her.
Be a loving parent to yourself.
It is a special joy to communicate with your inner child
and rediscover his/her secrets.
Relive the beautiful memories of the past.
Experience again the moments of your greatest happiness.
Fill your heart with these memories.
Fill your heart with peace, love, harmony, and serenity,
and there will be no room for anything else.

Within your spiritual heart you can talk to God
and commune with him.
Praise him, pray with him, petition him,
and do not be afraid.

Ask him to guide you, to inspire you,
to give you the strength to fulfill your creativity
and to give you the perseverance to continue,
even at times when you feel tired
and you want to quit.
"Do not let your heart be troubled."
Create a shield that makes your heart impermeable
to thoughts of envy, jealousy, hostility,
and all other negative emotions.
Let your heart be pure and simple.
Fill your heart with the spiritual values
of friendship, love, companionship,
and feed these values daily
in the spiritual garden of your mind.
The healing of your physical heart lies primarily
in the healing of your spiritual heart.
Clearing the channels of spirituality
is equivalent to opening wide the arteries
that feed your physical heart.
Keep these spiritual channels clear,
free from negative thoughts and feelings.
Allow yourself to communicate with your heart;
in turn, you will be able to touch the hearts
and lives of others.

Finally, your heart is the center of love.
Within your heart resides a spiritual flame
that is always burning.
Kahlil Gibran observes that the power to love
is God's greatest gift to humankind;

*for it will never be taken away
from the blessed one who loves.*
Love lies in the spiritual heart,
  not in the body,
  and stimulates our better self
  to welcome gifts of divine love.
Love is the only flower that grows and blossoms
  without the aid of seasons.

CHAPTER TWO

Coming to Grips with Heart Disease

"If you bring forth what is within you,
what you bring forth will save you.
If you do not bring forth what is within you,
what you do not bring forth will destroy you."
—JESUS (GOSPEL OF THOMAS)

GIVING IN TO DISEASE

We have all experienced disease and illness—there is a difference between the two. Disease is a malfunction of the body. Illness is how this malfunction reveals itself to us.

In the course of my life, I have seen that one's psychological and spiritual responses to a disease are often as important as the disease that the person happens to have. In my experience, not everybody responds to disease in the same way. There are patients who passively accept the diagnosis of the disease with resignation and denial. They blame outside forces for their destiny. The bottom line is that they do not want to change.

They come to the office carrying an imaginary bag, with all the medical problems they have suffered in their life. When they reach the doctor's desk they dump the bag. They look for a comfortable chair and say, "Doc, do what you have to do. Take care of it." Sometimes it is possible to do something; sometimes it is too late. Here's an example of such a patient—this comes from an actual interview:

Dr. Cortis: "Tell me about yourself. What happened?"

Patient: "Well, there isn't much to it. I was making dinner yesterday, something my wife likes, cabbage rolls. I was a cook in the navy. I set the table—my wife is an invalid. I ate five of them. An hour later I got a stabbing pain in my left side. It startled me. Tears came to my eyes. After about fifteen seconds it went away. I said to myself, 'Well, it's only gas pains from the cabbage.'

"While I was doing the dishes, I got another one. This time I went down on both knees. I had tears in my eyes again and I said, 'This is not right!'

"I stayed on my hands and knees and crawled to the pantry and reached for a bottle of Courvoisier. I poured myself a double shot thinking that whiskey is good for something like this. I sat there for about fifteen minutes. I didn't tell my wife.

"When I told my wife, she started to give me hell. We walked back to the kitchen. The whole room began to spin. The table was moving. My face fell down right on my plate. I blacked out. I tried to get up but I fell against the sink. I fell again and crawled to my

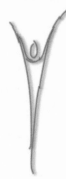

*E*xceptional heart patients have much to teach us about caring for our heart. These are people who are open to the spiritual dimension of their heart and face the fears and challenges of life and death head on. Death is the ultimate change in your life. You can use your heart intelligence to live life fully and prepare for it.

bedroom. Before I lay down I blacked out again. That was all I remembered.

"Later my wife told me that my sons came and dragged me to the car. We came to the emergency room here. I don't remember too much—some woman banging on my chest. I would have punched her if she was a guy. That hurt. The next thing I know I'm in the intensive care unit. I am asking everyone what happened and nobody wants to tell me anything. Now I feel I can play eighteen holes of golf.

"In cold weather, I can feel a drawing in the middle of my chest. I take nitroglycerin. That stops the pain.

"I had another heart attack about fifteen years ago. I used to smoke two to three packs a day then, working as a painter. I was flying to Houston, Texas. We were playing cards and all of a sudden, bingo, I blacked out. They told me I had a light stroke?

"The second one I had was a little stronger. I was having lunch one day and began to have this nauseating feeling. I got dizzy. I went home early. I was dizzy but I was able to walk across the street, get my car, and drive very fast to my home. Then I hit my fence and blacked out.

"The doctor told me I'm too fat: 'You got your warning; now you have to behave.' About five years ago I was playing golf. On the third hole my knees went out; I got dizzy and nauseated.

"I walk too fast and get shortness of breath, but only in cold weather. Also, when I pick up something heavy I feel it again.

"My brother died after his third heart attack. This scares the hell out of me!"

Dr. Cortis: "Well, my impression is that the pains may be coming from narrowing of the arteries within the heart. Let's find out once and for all, instead of guessing."

Patient: "When can I go home? I have to take care of my wife. She misses me. This is the worst thing that could happen—that I wind up in the hospital and she is at home helpless."

I share this interview with you because this person is a good example of the kind of patient I and other cardiologists see every day. He is our enigma. Despite repeated episodes of nausea, dizziness, shortness of breath, drawing pains in his chest which require nitroglycerin, his knees collapsing, blacking out, running into the fence with his car, collapsing into his dinner plate, having to crawl on his hands and knees, and finally being dragged to the emergency room where resuscitation measures are required, he wants to know when he can go home! He is worried about his wife, yes; but himself, no. He seems oblivious to himself, to his precarious hold on life. It's the "third" heart attack that "scares the hell" out of him. He simply has no clue to the deadly seriousness of his problem.

THE SECOND GROUP of patients are the obedient consumers. These are the A students of medicine. They obey the physician's order but they take no initiative. And they usually have an average outcome.

The third category, however, I classify as exceptional patients. These are individuals who focus on how healthy they are, not on how sick they are. They concentrate on living life rather than prolonging life. They see their heart disease as a challenge, as an opportunity to broaden their knowledge and awareness. While they might well have realistic fears for the future, they make a conscious choice to respond to their situation in a proactive way and take full responsibility. They look deeply into their heart and find the courage and perseverance to make the necessary changes to bring their lives into balance.

Exceptional heart patients do not always obey doctors' orders. In fact, they often cause their doctors a good deal of trouble by questioning their advice, refusing to go along with their prescribed treatment, or seeking second opinions. They demand a great deal of information about their condition. They want their doctors to serve as advisors and consultants, not as authorities. They insist on making the final decisions themselves.

Many employ some form of diet, exercise, meditation, spiritual involvement, and the power of love.

I am reminded of the experience of Mildred, a young woman who had developed bone cancer at the age of twelve and which resulted in her having one leg amputated. As a child she underwent radiation and chemotherapy. To further complicate her condition, she developed a heart problem that demanded a heart transplant at the age of eighteen.

This experience was enough to have destroyed anybody. Still, when I interviewed the patient over the phone, I heard a wonderful voice, full of life and enthusiasm. Not only did she recover and even get married later on, she was also working and raising a family. When I asked how she said, "I never give up." This is an exceptional person.

MYRON is another exceptional person. He is eighty-one years old, tall, bald, and has blue eyes and a gentle smile. He speaks softly. Myron had a large abdominal aortic aneurysm, a dilata-tion of the aorta. When I went to see him, he was lying down peacefully with his wife seated in the corner opposite the bed. She was holding her purse and her expression was that of tiredness. I explained the seriousness of the situation, but his face was calm and steady. He and his wife both told me: If it will happen, it will happen—but no surgery. What amazes me is that they both understood that it was a life-threatening illness. But they didn't fear death. They preferred to take their lives in their hands and accept all responsibility.

I saw Myron again in ICU the following morning; his vital signs were stable. His lack of fear and peaceful acceptance of his natural destiny delayed his reuniting with God for several years.

ONE MORE story. I was invited to a hospital in Nebraska to give a seminar. One lady attending the seminar shared with me the fact that her husband was waiting for a heart transplant, that he had been waiting for ten weeks. She asked me to see him.

When I entered his room, I realized that the patient's heart was connected to a mechanical heart that was performing the pumping action for him. As his wife introduced me to him, he made the attempt to sit up—he could bend just a little bit from the waist—and we shook hands. He was a relatively young man, maybe in his forties, intelligent face, powerful handshake. He still had all the energy of youth within his body, but his heart had been affected by several heart attacks. I wished him the best, and I touched his feet as I was leaving.

I was affected by what must have been going through the mind of the patient. First of all, he had to wait for somebody else to die in order to receive an organ transplant. Then, it required a profound faith to trust that a compatible donor would be found and that the surgery would be successful.

DEATH AND THE CARDIAC PATIENT

The fear of death is an extremely important concern for all of us. It is also a critical matter for cardiac patients. In essence, every new chest pain may signal the onset of another heart attack, maybe a worse one than before. So fear haunts cardiac patients because they are inclined to look at the heart, not as a powerful muscle able to recover, but as a broken vase that needs to be repaired and protected until it breaks again, and this time forever. They shy away from discussing the issue with their physician. Maybe they feel ashamed to experience the fear of death and they deny themselves the expression of this emotion.

In essence, it's like there's a hole in our heart. People treat it like a taboo: don't discuss it, we'll handle it ourselves. Even as a physician it's a hard question to ask. I have had the experience, paradoxically, of offending patients by inquiring what their feelings were about dying. They turned the question back on me: Why are you asking me this? Am I close to dying?

Elisabeth Kübler-Ross (*On Death and Dying*, Scribner's, 1997) is famous for her five psychological stages of dealing with one's own death: (1) Denial and isolation; (2) Anger, rage and envy; (3) Bargaining; (4) Depression; and (5) Acceptance. What should we do? First of all, ask ourselves the most important question: Are we living life to the fullest? Are we doing what we need to be doing? Second, plan and take action. And third, accept the reality of death. My wife Pia often says to our children: Bring me flowers while I can smell them.

With heart patients, death comes suddenly and unexpectedly. As a physician, I feel that I've let the person down, that I've let the family down. I was unable to predict the future, to see the outcome. The family may experience resentment, and sometimes the resentment comes to the fore in anger: the physician was late, he did not do enough, the treatment was inappropriate. The only way to avoid such situations is to face the issue, plan for contingencies, what ifs. I believe that in all instances physicians can be supportive.

I remember Frank, a patient whose blood pressure was about 60 and he was comatose. I asked the family members to join me in the CCU and the surge of love created a miracle. I saw his blood pressure rise on one of the monitors to 110. The patient had sensed the love surrounding him.

I always recommend that family members give permission to the dear one who is dying. Sometimes they hang on for a long time waiting for the family to give their consent.

I remember another patient, Neal, who was dying of cancer. I had the idea of asking him to recall moments from his childhood or teenage years. He began to describe his farm, the experience of playing with his brother, and riding horses. His eyes were smiling. He was happy remembering the beautiful moments of his life, even if the family was not around.

ON DEATH AND DYING

Death is a natural part of life. We can ignore it or we can face it and change our attitude. We can make use of this life while we still have time and know that when we die it will be without remorse. If we refuse to accept death now, we will not be able to live our lives fully. If we are prepared, there is a tremendous hope in life and in death.

Why do we live in fear of death? Because we wish to live and to go on living. Death in our eyes signifies the end to everything we hold familiar. The deepest reason we are terrified by death is because we don't know who we are. We believe only in our personal identity: our family, our job, our friends.

Sogyal Rinpoche wrote (*The Tibetan Book of Living and Dying*, HarperSanFrancisco, 1994) that "we live for what is always out of reach." Our thirst for survival in the future makes us incapable of living in the present. The pace of our lives is so hectic that the last thing we have time to think about is death. We confound ourselves with goods and comforts. All our time and energy is exhausted keeping everything as safe as possible. And so our lives move on unless a serious illness or accident takes us.

The Tibetan word for body is *lü*, which means "something you leave behind." It is helpful to imagine our own death: the sensations, the grief of our loved ones, the pain, the helplessness, and the realization of what we have left undone. Death is real and unpredictable.

We should ask ourselves, How much have I understood life and death? "The main goal in life is to learn to love other people and to acquire knowledge," says Rinpoche.

Let me share with you an experience. Years ago my brother died of cancer of the esophagus. We had been very close for a long time. We had many dreams. One of them was getting together every summer, and we did that for twenty-five years. Often he came to the States to spend additional time with me. And we planned on being together in retirement to spend time on the beach discussing and sharing feelings, opening our hearts like you can only do with a brother.

Unexpectedly, he died. What I learned in his generosity to me was that I began to ask myself, *If I had six months to live, would I continue to do what I am doing now?* The answer was, *Of course not.* I am making the decision now to sell my practice and let my spirit tell me what to do, such as writing about the spirituality of the heart, teaching and increasing the knowledge of the God within me.

This is what I have learned. What does it have to do with the heart? Within our heart we have to ask ourselves the key question. Is the life we are living now the one we want to live? What do we do with the material goods we are accumulating? We keep acquiring things as if we are going to be here forever.

Consider that one day our heart will stop beating. Our physical life will stop. This requires an element of preparation, and all of us have to be prepared. The best time to get ready is while we are well and our body is functioning properly, not when a catastrophic illness compels us to confront the issue.

The final question is to ask our heart how we want to be remembered. What do we want done when we die? Do we want to be buried or cremated? Take the initiative of planning these moments and save your family and loved ones the unpleasantness of having to do it for you.

I have some pictures of myself in the attic and I was looking at them, smiling and relaxing. I thought a new approach to death would be to make a celebration of your life. What you have done. How you have contributed. Moments of joy. What would you like to share with others as you enter the spiritual domain and a new life in the arms of God?

"The purpose of life on earth is to achieve union with our enlightened nature." Our society is dedicated to the celebration of the ego and quick fixes. It is our spiritual heart that shows us the path that is most meaningful to us and contains the secret of our destination. By tuning ourselves to this divine organ we avoid becoming a spiritual tourist. Rinpoche writes: "Never getting anywhere? Choose one path and follow it." Our spiritual heart is the answer.

ACTIVATING YOUR BIOLOGICAL FORCE TO PREVENT AND HEAL HEART DISEASE

You have a very profound healing power within yourself, within your body. The primary component of this healing power is awareness. And awareness can be achieved by anybody. I was not aware of this spiritual reality until I had been practicing for many years. Now, I see that most of our problems originate in our minds;

most of our diseases are diseases of self, brought on by the self.

When I say that disease is a self-induced experience I mean that it is a result of a maladjustment to life or to a life situation, an inordinate amount of stress or an inappropriate response to stimuli. Ultimately, the origin of the disease is in the mind. This is why treating illness with medicine alone does not heal. It only provides a temporary solution; it only addresses the physical manifestation of the problem.

We all have the power to heal ourselves. The only problem is that the power can remain unused for our entire lives if we do not become aware of it. How can you evoke the healing power? First, be aware that this power exists. Open yourself to the spiritual dimension of yourself, the dimension that is always free from disease. Open yourself to becoming a self-healer. Be aware of your body and its needs.

Second, believe that you can get better. Your faith is fundamental for healing and your spiritual heart is the primary source.

THE HEART HAS ITS OWN INTELLIGENCE

The heart has always been pictured as the center of our emotions and of our feelings. When we imagine the heart, many attributes come to mind: a happy heart, a sad heart, a joyful heart, and a loving heart. We feel in our heart, we see in our heart, we know in our heart, we expect in our heart. But is the heart only the center of our emotions and feelings?

Is there anything more to this spiritual organ? I have an image of Jesus that comes from the Catholic tradition. I see superimposed on his chest the image of a heart surrounded by a crown. It is an image of the Sacred Heart of Jesus. Jesus has been depicted for centuries with this image of the heart to represent his love for humankind.

Within the heart we find the deepest values we treasure, in essence, the core of our being, the individuality of our own spirit. I also believe that in addition to our memories the heart is the center of our wisdom.

The heart has its own intelligence. Most of the time we are guided by the intelligence of the mind. The work of the mind is to look into our memory bank and locate past experiences in reference to the present. The message then comes loud and clear: don't do this, don't do that; do this, do that; trust, do not trust. As Deepak Chopra says, the intelligence of the mind is guided by the ego, that part of us that is always in search of power, control, and approval. There will never be enough to satisfy the ego, which by nature is independent and insatiable.

The driving force of the ego is fear of losing what one has. The counterpart of the ego is the spiritual heart, which is driven by love. If the heart is the center of our authenticity, of our affection, of our deepest desire, if within the heart we can find the center of ourselves, why not use the intelligence of the heart to be guided throughout life?

Just for curiosity, think of a situation and examine your mental response. I did it thinking of my father's death. I was not there when he died—he died in Italy—and I experienced guilt for a long time. I was wracking my mind for answers to that situation. And my mind was loading me up with guilt: I could have done this and I could have done that.

It was too late to change what happened, but when I addressed the same question to my heart the answers were completely different. I learned that my father loved me. He loved me immensely. When he was dying he was calling my name.

The intelligence of the heart is different from that of the mind. The mind seeks victories. The heart seeks solutions. The mind seeks independence. The heart seeks connectedness. The mind is judgmental. The heart is forgiving. It is clear that material matters drive the mind; the heart is driven by spiritual values. It is as if God guides the heart.

ASK YOUR HEART

The eyes of your spiritual heart are enlightened. The challenge is for you to use your heart intelligence. Here's an exercise that will get you started.

Exercise

Look back over your life. Remember an experience that in your mind was painful, a time when you judged yourself harshly. Now review this same episode from the perspective of your heart, with the eyes of your heart. What words would come from your heart? Open yourself to the healing power of your spiritual heart.

MAKE PEACE WITH CHANGE

As we look back over our lives, we see so many changes. One change after another. Some of the most difficult episodes in our lives have involved making a change. What is it about change that represents such a challenge? Think about how you address change in your life. Are you a reactor or an instigator? Do you take charge or follow the flow? Do you recognize the need for change or do you strive to hold on to what you have? Can you reach into the stillness and peace of your spiritual heart to overcome the sense of fear or loss that often accompanies a major change?

Meditation

Everything in life changes.
 Nature changes.
 The seasons change.
 Our bodies change.
 Our minds change.
Everything around us is in constant change.
There is a universal law that is immutable:
 Everything changes;
 nothing is permanent.
Why then do we work so hard
 to keep ourselves and our possessions as safe as possible
 by avoiding change at all cost?
It is because any change,
 any mutation,
 is a challenge to our control.
The driving force in our mind,
 our ego,
 fears the loss of control.
As the spiritual heart becomes our center of reference,
 we accept change,
 we empower ourselves,
 we see through the eyes of God.

CHAPTER THREE

The Heart
As Spiritual Organ

*"The God you are seeking is the God
at the center of your being."*
—CARLETON WHITEHEAD

MORE THAN A MUSCLE

S uppose I were to ask you "Which part of your body do you
identify with the most?" Would it be your liver? Your
kidney? Your brain? Your big toe? I imagine the question would
make you laugh because most likely you don't identify with any
of these. Whether you realize it or not, the part of your body
that you most identify with, that you realize represents your
true self, your higher self, is your heart.

If you doubt the truth of this statement, imagine that you
have just received some very good news. Where do you feel the
excitement and elation? In your heart. And where do you feel
the pain of bad news? In the same place, of course, in your
heart. We feel the emotions of love most strongly, first of all, in
our heart.

A number of rather well-known sayings reinforce the wisdom of this truth. Certainly you've heard people speak of their "heart of hearts," a phrase that Shakespeare used. As for the primacy of the heart over the mind, consider Shakespeare again: "The head is not more native to the heart" (*Hamlet*). Noted French philosopher Blaise Pascal (1623–1662) gives us this one: "The heart has its reasons which are quite unknown to the head." And François de la Rochefoucauld (1614–1680) adds: "Intellect is always fooled by the heart."

These sayings express a real truth, one that we all recognize instinctively. After all, the most profound qualities that we seek in life are all to be found in the heart—love, inner peace, happiness, humility, compassion. Yet our scientific, "rational" world insists that the heart is, in fact, simply one of many organs in the body, with no special characteristics. I remember a transplant surgeon who once told a recovering transplant patient, "The heart is only a muscle. A stupid muscle."

I was so shocked I couldn't find words to speak. How could he say that? I wondered. And how could he say it to a transplant patient who had just received the precious gift of a new heart? The patient knew the truth, however. He replied, "I know that's not true, because since the transplant I have had feelings I did not have before."

As this patient instinctively knew, the heart has its own memories, often different than those of the "mind." If you doubt this, visit a place you have not seen since childhood, and observe how your heart responds with a faster, stronger beat.

My own experiences with transplant patients further demonstrate the reality of the heart's memory. I have inter-viewed dozens of people with new hearts, and a significant

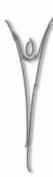

The heart is more than a muscle. If you doubt this, you need only speak with some heart transplant patients. These individuals have a special insight into the wisdom of the heart. There are exercises you can use to determine for yourself how attuned you are to your spiritual heart. And the writings of all our major religious traditions will point you in that direction.

number of them believe that a part of their donor's life has been transferred to them along with the heart. Although I cannot prove it, I do believe that the heart has memory cells, and that they are transplanted along with the heart. The following is an edited excerpt from a typical interview with one of these remarkable heart transplant patients:

Dr. Cortis: "Mr. Smith, what led up to your heart transplant?"

Mr. Smith: "Well, my diagnosis was viral cardiomyopathy. I was being treated by my GP for what I thought was the flu and bronchitis and then overnight, it seemed, I filled up and ended up with end-stage congestive heart failure. Within two hours of walking into the hospital they put me on a balloon pump and told my wife I needed a heart transplant, if I could survive the next three days because of the liquid that had built up in me. My kidneys had basically shut down. They had me frozen on ice and paralyzed, but they finally got them to work again. I was evaluated as a status one case.

"Basically, *status one* means you could die within forty-eight hours and you're put at the top of the list for transplants. . . . I had basically three problems at that time, cardiogenic shock, viral cardiomyopathy, and congestive heart failure. They found out I was 98 percent blocked over all my coronary arteries, plus I had a heavy virus they couldn't identify, which made me run a very high fever.

"They basically told me I had a hundred percent chance of not surviving, but if we can find a heart donor you might. I ended up being on a balloon pump for sixteen days, which set some kind of record. On about the eleventh day there was an opportunity for a transplant, but after I was prepped for surgery and moved downstairs, they called and said the left ventricle was not good; the heart was not good. That was the worst day of my life.

"The next opportunity came five days later and they told me my chances were fifty-fifty. So I went to surgery. After surgery, I went through the normal recovery process and on the seventh day they put me out of the hospital. The total hospital stay was twenty-five days. It was like a month from hell."

Dr. Cortis: "You describe it as if it were yesterday."

Mr. Smith: "I am out five years this month. The reason I describe it so clearly is because I donate a great deal of my time seeing those who are waiting for transplants and those who are being evaluated for transplants. I talk their language and I can answer a lot of questions. You need to have a nonphysician talk to them because they don't always trust the medical profession and there are a lot of things they won't ask a doctor which they will ask me.

"I spend the other half of my time, which is probably the most important to me, speaking to medical professionals. I speak in all the hospitals, to every group from neurosurgery to ER to physicians and nurses. . . ."

Dr. Cortis: "Have you had any unusual experiences after the transplant? Any changes in personality?"

Mr. Smith: "Well, not any personality changes, but my wife said I seem to like dancing more, and colors, and stuff like that."

Dr. Cortis: "Like selections of taste."

Dr. Smith: "I would say the selection of clothes. I am fairly conservative and I was a lot less conservative in my clothes. I didn't really change a lot as far as music. I think the second time around you tend to recognize things more and take more time. I am an A-type personality, even in my business. Right now, the biggest change that has happened to me is that I've gone from being ultramaterialistic to the complete reverse: what can I give back to society? How can I help? That's certainly connected with the fact that they saved my life and whatever I can do to help someone else I would do it. But I've also taken the stance that nobody is going to rush me to get me to do things anymore. Time is important but it is not important enough to get myself all exercised about something. So that is a change I also went through."

Dr. Cortis: "A change in personal growth."

Mr. Smith: "Yes, of course, you know, when you come out of a transplant you really have no concept of what it's going to be like. A lot of transplants have been in bad shape for twenty years and unable to do anything and for them to have a transplant is a miraculous change. For me it certainly was a miraculous change, but I'm always trying to come back and do the same things. I am a lot more conscious of my health, my exercise. I run 5K races, which I never did before. I was a competitive person but I never did that. My drive to stay healthy is much much stronger."

Dr. Cortis: "Any other changes?"

Mr. Smith: "Not really. It took me three years to come to the point that I am not a sick person and that my going on with things is most important. The fact that I had a transplant is in the background now. I've reversed the direction there. I relate this experience all the time because I don't want to just sit and dwell on it. The only problems I really had afterward were accepting two things: one, that someone had to die in order for me to live, and two, that this organ is mine—it took me a year to get over this part of it."

Dr. Cortis: "And now in your consciousness you have accepted this?"

Mr. Smith: "Yes. It is mine."

Dr. Cortis: "I can sense that you are fully integrated."

JUMPERS

Here is another remarkable experience from a heart transplant patient named Michael:

Dr. Cortis: "Michael, you told me the story of what you experienced. Now there is something I want to ask you, if it is not too painful to remember, and that's about the out-of-body experiences you had during the time they were working on you before the transplant."

Michael: "I call them the "jumpers." My body, my face lifted up and went into the ceiling. I felt my body come off the table about eight inches, but my whole consciousness went into the ceiling itself, and then zoomed back down again. Then about four days later it happened again when they had to work on me again, you know, put the cables on me.

"What happened that time was that, as soon as I saw the cables coming toward me, all of a sudden my consciousness was in the corner of the room watching my body getting the stuff done to me."

Dr. Cortis: "That sounds incredible. You also told me that you experienced some kind of rejection, but then you got over it."

Michael: "Yes, that's right. What happened was that the soul of the person I got the heart from actually had the problem because the heart was still beating but there was no body. The body he knew was gone. This person had to go on to the next level but was lost because the shock came so quickly and death occurred—there was no adjustment period. And so this soul was wandering for a while. I met this shaman, this medicine man, who made contact with him and had a conversation. The shaman escorted him to another teacher who was awaiting him and he agreed to go with him."

Dr. Cortis: "I see."

Michael: "They couldn't knock out the rejection I was experiencing. I had fourteen biopsies, all minus 1A rejection. But the next week I went back and the negative rejection was gone."

Dr. Cortis: "That's fantastic."

A NEAR-DEATH EXPERIENCE

The following experience was related to me by a transplant patient by the name of Joseph.

Joseph: "My heart was hanging on to the slimmest of threads. The surgeons had been in to see me at about 4:30 P.M. with the results of five days of extensive testing, which explored all the options available to me. They seemed very discouraged. I wanted to ask them about their lack of enthusiasm, but I had been stuck in a prostrate position on my back with tubes extending from nearly every orifice. I was wondering how I could communicate since I wasn't able to speak.

"The morphine and dopomine had me flying high above the earth, cruising above the clouds, free from pain. At times, it felt as if a baby elephant was sitting on my chest preventing my lungs from expanding enough to fill with air. I was being challenged to gather all my strength and try to poke out my thoughts on a clipboard. I finally squeaked out, "What's up?" and the surgeons informed me of my near-hopeless predicament. They had placed me on the list as a transplant recipient with a status one rating because I was so near death.

"To keep me alive, they would have to give me a Novacor Left Ventricular Assist Device (a mechanical heart implanted below the diaphragm), which would do the job until a donor was found. This would be only the sixth or seventh procedure of this sort attempted in the world."

Dr. Cortis: "You must have been scared to death and overwhelmed with questions."

Joseph: "Did I have questions? How in the world could I have voiced them? All I could do was shake my head, yes or no. Granted, I was at a university medical center, one of the premier transplant centers in the country. Yet fear and terror rippled through my body with every other breath. Talk about being scared and frustrated. I preferred being out of this body as much as I could. There were several times I thought about flying off without returning. The sense of peace and tranquility I found in those clouds was quite seductive.

"There was the touch of a certain nurse, in the middle of the night, on my right hand, that immediately brought me back into consciousness. Did she see something on the monitors that was life-threatening that caused her to act so, as if she was calling on me to return? I needed to decide if I wanted to return to the world of the living. I needed to summon all my courage and strength to affirm life, even though the angel of death was right there summoning me to cross his threshold."

Dr. Cortis: "How did you cope?"

Joseph: "I lay there groping for breath, trying to hold on to a reason to continue. There was absolutely nothing I could do. I looked around my room and saw some of the many cards sent to me. I remembered being told that the switchboard operators were asking those who called about me to stop because I had had so many calls it made it impossible for the staff to answer all the queries and still perform their necessary duties. This was the first time in my life that I truly understood that there were many people who loved and cared about me being in their lives. The present reality brought me such understanding.

"I felt like I was wedged in a narrow rock opening of some unexplored cave. All I could do was lay back and surrender to the will of that which is beyond me. I could feel the prayers and hopes of all those dear friends surround and protect me. This gave me the strength to confront my fears.

"Once again, when I closed my eyes, I was lifted above the clouds, with the blue sky above and the white pillow clouds below. I was soaring. My arms were outstretched, acting as wings. I was moving quite fast, without any conscious direction or purpose, just accelerating beyond time and place. What a seductive feeling of contentment. Freedom and peace was overcoming me, alone but unafraid, for the first time in my life. Nothing to fear, not even myself.

"I zoomed back into my room a little after seven, when the surgeons returned. They had received word from the donor network that a heart had been located that matched my criteria."

RELYING ON OUR HEART INTELLIGENCE

Traditionally, we believe that we think with our heads, but that we experience love in our hearts. The reality is that we also think from the heart, through emotion and instinct, and the wisdom of the heart is often superior to that of the brain.

In the Book of Sirach (Ecclesiastes), the author writes: "God gives us the heart to think with, and the light in our heart is a spark of the divine heart." Although it may seem strange to *think* with the heart, the truth is that our heart has an intelligence of its own. In fact, the concept of wisdom is often connected with the heart in scripture and literature. In a very real way, we all think, speak, and reason with the heart, especially when in interaction with people we care about.

We also rely on the heart's intelligence whenever we make any important decision. For example, no matter how carefully you may weigh all options, ultimately something serves to make you decide one way or another. In many if not most cases, this is your heart speaking, giving you the "feeling" that you should do one thing rather than another. Whether you realize this or not, you have consulted your heart as to the wisdom of the choices you are confronted with.

PUT YOURSELF ON THE BRAIN/HEART SPECTRUM

The following columns of words are inspired by Paul Pearsall (*The Heart's Code*, Broadway Books, 1998). They show different qualities of the brain and the heart. There are no right words and there are no wrong words. They are qualities. You will relate naturally to one side or the other, and it may change from left to right.

Exercise

Rearrange the order of these columns of "opposites" in the order of their importance to you. Some words will obviously mean more to you than others. Pick these first. Start by identifying the ten words that best describe you. Use the two columns on the right. How many are on the "Heart" side? Are you more brain oriented or heart oriented? After you have given this some time, come back to the exercise and pick the next ten important words.

Opposite Qualities:		Words That Best Describe You:	
Brain	**Heart**	**Brain**	**Heart**
Victories	Solutions		
Power	Peace		
Control	Serenity		
Approval	Balance		
Fear	Love		
Thinks	Feels		
Achievements	Meaning		
Satisfaction	Fulfillment		

61

Think with your brain	Think with your heart	_____	_____
Looks for cure	Looks for healing	_____	_____
Remembers	Forgets	_____	_____
Unforgiving	Forgives	_____	_____
Imperfections	Perfection	_____	_____
Material	Spiritual	_____	_____
Fear worries	Peace, serenity	_____	_____
Strength	Understanding	_____	_____
Malicious	Innocent	_____	_____
Hard logic	Blind faith	_____	_____
Domain	Freedom	_____	_____
Heartless	Heartfelt	_____	_____
Success	Connection	_____	_____
Doing	Being	_____	_____
Type A brain	Type B heart	_____	_____
Independence	Connectedness	_____	_____
Separation	Bonding	_____	_____
"Needs to have a blast"	"Needs to have a bond"	_____	_____
Territorial— "me-mine"	Nonterritorial— "Ours"	_____	_____
Impatient	Patient	_____	_____
Just do it	Let it be	_____	_____
Control	Be limited	_____	_____

Do your own thing	Do our thing	_____	_____
Defensive	Agreeable	_____	_____
Negative	Congenial	_____	_____
Hostile	Harmonious	_____	_____
Ego—self	Spirit—otherness	_____	_____
Pessimistic	Optimistic	_____	_____
Selfish	Altruistic	_____	_____
Primarily reactive	Contemplative	_____	_____
Maintenance system	Feeling system	_____	_____
Knows it all	Open to finding out	_____	_____

THE SPIRITUAL HEART IN SACRED WRITINGS

What we may feel instinctively, that the heart is much more than just a bodily organ, has been revealed over and over in the sacred writings of many traditions. These writings demonstrate that the heart is indeed the place where life originates, and that our spiritual qualities are directly related to the quality of our heart.

In the Christian Bible, for example, the heart is mentioned 592 times in 550 verses. It is beyond the scope or intent of this book to catalogue all the different ways the heart has been mentioned in sacred writing, but I recommend reading some of these verses whenever you feel a special need to get in touch with your heart. Here are some of my favorite sacred references to the heart, and a little personal commentary on them:

- *Lord, you made us, Lord, for yourself, and our heart is restless until it rests in you.* (SAINT AUGUSTINE)

  Each of us has this in common: that we are looking for joy and happiness in life. I firmly believe that each of us, whether we realize it or not, is in search of God, or whatever image we have of the divine. When the search is over, and we find God, so do we find happiness. After all, it was God who gave us the commandment: "You shall love the Lord your God with your whole heart" (Matthew 22:38).

  Other traditions as well recognize this truth: In *The Mystic Heart* (New World Library, 1999), author Wayne Teasdale quotes the great Native American leader Black Elk, who said: "The heart is a sanctuary at the center of which there is a little space wherein the Great Spirit dwells, and this is the eye. This is the eye of the Great Spirit by which he sees all things, and through which we see him. If the heart is not pure the Great Spirit cannot be seen."

  When you talk to the Divine, you communicate from your heart. The heart is actually a stepping stone that allows us to transcend ourselves, our human nature, and communicate with the spirit within.

- *More than all else, keep watch over your heart, since here are the wellsprings of life.* (PROVERBS 4:23)

This quote reaffirms that the heart is the source of all our feelings and emotions. It is the heart alone that can guide us in what we do and how we behave.

- *The life of the body is a tranquil heart.*　　(PROVERBS 4:30).

This saying emphasizes that true health lies within a peaceful heart. In modern medicine we focus too much on traditional, technological means of healing, and tend to ignore the spiritual aspects, which would lead to true and lasting healing. Another verse reaffirms this truth: "A glad heart is excellent medicine" (Proverbs 17:22).

- *Worry makes a man's heart heavy. A kindly word makes it glad.*　　(PROVERBS)

The prophets were ahead of modern medicine in recognizing that negative emotions can have a bad effect on our health. Numerous writings in all sacred traditions caution against hardening of the heart, or closing it off. When we become self-centered and forget that we are in this world to serve others, we betray ourselves as well.

Whenever you experience negative attitudes, such as hatred, hostility, or the desire to cause harm to others, go within your heart and ask for direction to a positive outlook on your life.

- *Let these words, I urge you, be written on your heart.*
　　(DEUTERONOMY 6:6)

The Word is very near to you. It is in your heart and in your mouth. (DEUTERONOMY 30:14)

In these and other biblical verses we are invited to meditate within our heart. In a later chapter, we'll examine meditation in more detail. But the wisdom of countless religious traditions emphasizes that the heart is an integral part of any prayerful or meditative practice.

- *I shall give you a new heart and put a new spirit in you.*
(EZEKIEL 36:24-27).

The spirit the prophet is referring to is the spirit of love and openness, essential for communicating with God as well as with other humans. I believe that true communication is possible only when we speak from the heart. Think about it. Most often when we "communicate" with others, we express opinions and judgments. When we open our hearts and express our true feelings, however, real communication can occur and we can achieve intimacy. The heart in essence expresses the inner core of a person.

- *Your body does not perceive what your heart perceives.*
(SAINT AUGUSTINE).

He invites us to return to our heart to become enlightened. A great part of the wisdom of the heart comes from its purpose as the seat of all love. It can help us learn to realize that happiness in our life relies on our ability to love; to love others, to love ourselves, and to love the Divine.

- *The love of God has been poured into their hearts.*

(ROMANS 5:5)

Whether we realize it or not, our hearts are full of love— the love of the Divine. Our mission in life is to be of service to others, to be spiritual missionaries guided by our hearts.

According to the aforementioned Blaise Pascal, the heart is the guide that helps us to see our moral and religious destiny. The heart's own knowledge, says Pascal, is "direct, intuitive, and flexible."

It is in our heart that the solutions to our problems lie. In our heart alone can we hear the voice of the Divine. Within our heart we find everything that we are.

- *If your heart is pure, then all things in your world are pure.*

(RYOKAN ZEN POETRY)

All traditions aspire to purity of heart. Jesus said, "Blessed are the pure in heart," while Proverbs affirms that "God loves the pure in heart." I feel that purity is primarily a matter of humbleness combined with a true desire to seek the truth.

- *The mind creates the abyss, and the heart crosses it.*

(SRI NISARGADATTA)

This saying by a famous Indian mystic clearly demonstrates the gap between the "rational" mind and the loving heart.

We all know the saying, "Nothing is good or bad; thinking only makes it so." It is the thinking mind that creates most of our troubles, after all, by providing worries, excuses, and resentments. Whereas, if we simply accept with an open and loving heart, we can overcome nearly any obstacle.

I'm sure you know people who can turn any setback into a terrible tragedy, while others accept life's greatest burdens lightly and with loving acceptance.

ASSESSING YOUR SPIRITUAL HEART

We have within ourselves this divine organ, the source of our life. And signals from our heart have the deepest meaning, what I call "heart hints." These heart hints are like light in moments of darkness, a pathway to our health and healing.

Meditation

Accessing your spiritual heart is as simple as just being.
All of us have this treasure within ourselves,
  whether or not we are aware of it.
The spiritual heart offers us all the wealth we need.
It is a spiritual banquet
  where the host and the guest
  are the same person—you.
It is a domain of timelessness animated by love;
  a return to naturalness,
  simplicity,
  and authenticity.

In the spiritual heart
    you are in the eternal present.
You are the universe itself,
    and the universe is you.
In your spiritual heart
    you and God are one.
You discover the purpose of life
    to become all that you are.
In your spiritual heart
    you find freedom to be.
As you see through the eyes of your heart,
    you will learn that you are pure love.

CHAPTER FOUR

Taking Your Spiritual Inventory

Let us swing wide all the doors and windows
of our hearts on their rusty hinges
so we may learn how to open in love.

Let us see the light in the other and honor it
so we may lift one another on our shoulders
and carry each other along.

Let holiness move in us
so we may pay attention to its small voice
and give ourselves fully with both hands.
—DAWNA MARKOVA

SEEKING A SPIRITUAL OUTLOOK

Religion can have many meanings. But for many, being religious simply means practicing or belonging to a specific religious tradition. Spirituality, on the other hand, implies an active search for the divine, as well as for meaning. It is only within our hearts that true spirituality can be fulfilled.

Religion is a set of rules about the spiritual, a bridge to the spiritual. But spirituality is more. It is your personal relationship with the Divine.

In my life I have found three kinds of spiritual outlook:

- the voluntarily spiritually deprived, those who are cynical and don't believe in spirituality;

- the obedient religious, those who go to church and attend church functions, but see God as a punishing force; and

- the true seekers, those who realize that everything in the universe is of a spiritual nature and seek the Divine in order to nourish themselves and others.

I believe that only members of the third group—the true seekers—are able to call upon their spiritual strength to prevent and overcome illness and to live meaningful and fulfilled lives, no matter what outside forces beat at them.

STRESS

One of the major stumbling blocks to our spiritual life is stress. Stress creates a sense of urgency and anxiety that affects our heart and our entire existence. What is stress? Stress is a condition of the way our mind and body adapt to change. Among the most basic of human needs is the urge to control ourselves and others all the time. Stress is linked to control.

Stress can come on suddenly, or it can develop over a long term. Short-term stress is often prompted by an unexpected event that is perceived as a challenge to our control. This

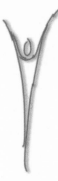

S pirituality is your personal relationship with the Divine. One of the major stumbling blocks to your spiritual life is stress. This is the sense of urgency and anxiety we place on ourselves at times when we perceive a challenge to our control over life. You can overcome stress in your life by being in tune with your spiritual heart, by becoming a spiritually healthy person.

creates an alarm reaction characterized by fear, perspiration, and rapid heartbeat. Long-term stress, however, is experienced as a sense of failure or entrapment, created by forces over which we have lost control. Under these circumstances there are bodily changes, such as an increase in gastric acid, with possible ulcers, a depression of our immune system, together with a reduced production of sex hormones. The affected person tends to avoid work and is prone to accidents.

It is important to realize that stress in and of itself is not the culprit. It is not something that assaults us from the outside, like a virus. Rather, it is a condition that we create within ourselves. The problem lies in the way we perceive stress and how we react when we feel we are outside our "comfort zone."

Handling stress means controlling the fear, anxiety and despair we experience in situations we find stressful. When we realize that we create the feelings and emotions in response to challenges to our control, we become aware that we have a choice! If our reaction is negative and disempowering, we are the only one who can change this reaction. Blaming people and circumstances for our response to stress is a waste of time. So is trying to change them.

Instead, we must focus on changing the way we react. The key point is changing ourselves. Say to yourself: "My reaction to stress is my choice. I am responsible. If I don't like my self-defeating response to stress, I can choose to change it. It's up to me! Viewed in this manner, stress becomes a learning experience and an opportunity to know yourself better.

Gary Zukav (*The Heart of the Soul: Emotional Awareness*, with Linda Francis, Fireside, 2002) defines stress as a resistance to your life: disliking your job, your present circumstances, even yourself. Stress is proportional to the degree of your resistance. This inner conflict deprives you of emotional energy. The solution lies, Zukav says, in giving up resistance and accepting reality as such. Acceptance generates the same calmness we experience when we make a decision. As we accept our life we can direct our energy toward changes we need to make. It is like transcending yourself and gaining a higher vision that leads to problem solving.

Stress, in essence, can be viewed as a friend. It points us in the direction we need to work on so that we become more patient and self supportive and gain understanding. If we could direct the energy we waste handling stress toward our spiritual life, we would vastly simplify our existence.

STRESS AND LIFE EXPERIENCES

We link stress to life experiences that have left deep impressions on our mind and soul. Allow me to share with you one such experience. Almost every summer I would visit my mother at her beach house. One morning, I decided with my older sister Delia to go to the cemetery and pay a visit to my father's grave. In the late afternoon, a phone call brought us back to the village. My mother had fallen sick.

I ran to the house where I found several friends and relatives. My brother Nello just looked at me and shook his head. When I got inside, I saw my mother lying in bed. She was wearing the blue dress with flowers that I had brought her from Chicago. Her face was serene and peaceful, her eyes closed, a white band around her chin and forehead. I put my arms around her and hugged and kissed her. In tears I cried, "Mother, mother, don't leave me!" I kissed her hair, her eyes, and her face, as if I could give life back to her. She was immobile. She was gone.

It was like I was dreaming. My brother Nello and my sisters Delia and Rita were in tears. We hugged each other saying, "Mother is dead; she is gone forever."

I slept in a room next to her and frequently went to tell her how much I missed her, and how much I loved her. In the afternoon, two people from the funeral home brought the casket and together with them we transferred her body into the coffin. Her body was stiff; she was very light and cold. There was a rosary in her hands.

Before these people came, I had spent much time with her, crying, hugging her over and over, and kissing her face. I begged her forgiveness for not giving her as much love as she deserved. I had moved to the States and left her twenty years before, after she had raised me and afforded me the opportunity to become a physician. I knew that she had missed me. On many occasions she told me that she was hoping one day I would come back forever.

Before sealing the coffin, the two gentlemen from the funeral home put a pillow under her head and a long veil covering her entire body. One by one, we all kissed her for the last time.

Obviously, the experience of my mother's death had a great impact on me. I am sitting here now and remembering my mother. Just two days before her death, I was sitting next to her and holding her hand. I confessed to her how grateful I was to her for having raised me and for all the sacrifices she had made for me in her life, especially the one of letting me go forever. I asked her to look at me and I told her I loved her. Our eyes met and she gave me a long hug and a kiss. I am forever grateful for that opportunity to tell her these things I felt in my heart.

SPIRITUAL HEALTH

What are the attributes of a spiritually healthy person? These are highest on my list:

- Self-acceptance. Embracing all of ourself and our personality without reservations. The more we endorse ourselves, the easier it is to integrate our strengths and our weaknesses. We gain self-approval as we broaden our self-perception. We no longer identify ourselves with our job, for example; we are more than our work.

- Sense of self. Having a strong sense of self based upon self-acceptance and self-knowledge. Who we are is our foundation. The spiritual qualities we have been endowed with are the source of our strength.

- Authenticity. Being able to be ourselves naturally. We are most ourselves when our spirit shines unbounded. Allowing our soul to guide our lives to our own purpose is what makes us real.

- Responsibility. Accepting with dignity our mission and being accountable for ourselves. Responding to people and circumstances without blame reveals our measure of responsibility.

- Communicability. Being willing to open our heart and express our deepest feelings without judgment.

- The ability to love. Expressing love unconditionally, accepting affection from others, and achieving intimacy.

FINDING YOUR SPIRITUAL HEART

When you are separated from your heart, you are in a world driven by the ego. You become a victim of your feelings and are dominated by your senses. The world around you feels isolated and disconnected. You are in your spiritual heart when you are spontaneous and authentic, when your uniqueness shines unbounded. When you act as a real person, you are totally free from any conditioning to live through the ego.

I am attuned to my spiritual heart when I accept all of myself, when I trust the world, when I feel protected and guided by God. This is a sign of the presence of the spirit of God within.

When I sense that I am divinely inspired, I enter my spiritual heart.

TAKING A SPIRITUAL INVENTORY

This exercise is designed to put you in touch with your heart and give it a prominent place in your life, to tune in to your spiritual "heartbeat."

The following questions will get you started toward identifying where you are moving in your life and where your spirit wants you to go. As you consider them, other questions may present themselves and help you in defining your spiritual path. The end result will be to discover your greatest treasure: your spiritual heart and yourself

Exercise

1. *What makes you feel spiritual?*
2. *What does happiness mean to you?*
3. *When do you experience connectedness?*
4. *Which activities make you lose track of time altogether?*
5. *How have your life aspirations changed over the years?*
6. *What life events have prompted your spiritual growth?*
7. *How does your present lifestyle respond to your spiritual needs?*

INTIMACY WITH YOUR HEART

If only you knew what treasures your spiritual heart holds for you! It's time to open communication with the sanctuary of your soul. You need only be willing to receive the gifts of your heart.

Meditation

O Lord, open my heart
   to your compassion and wisdom.
Let your vision enlighten my vision.
Guide me.
Inspire me to serve you.
Fill my heart with kindness and compassion.
Open my heart, O Lord,
   to the infinity of your love.
Give me the perseverance
   to follow your path
   with patience and humility.
Give me the faith to believe
   that with you, O Lord,
   all things are possible.

CHAPTER FIVE

Fill Your Heart with Love

"A joyful heart is the inevitable result
of a heart burning with love."
—MOTHER TERESA

THE FORCE WITHIN

My older sister phoned recently to tell me her son was in love. His girlfriend is a physician studying cardiology. When I woke this morning, I couldn't take my mind off the memory of that conversation, because it so clearly spoke to me about how we feel inside when we are in love. It is a phenomenon that grabs the whole person. No question, when we are in love, we are cheerful and optimistic. We smile. We are happy. We are overcome with joy because, after so many years of waiting, we have finally found a soul mate to be our companion for life. I am absolutely sure about this. My sister's phone call brought the truth of it home to me so clearly.

Why do we know this? Because our heart tells us. When my nephew found this woman to love, he found his companion for life, his soul mate. Love is the fulfillment of all the dreams we harbor, of all the things two persons in love can do together: build a house, have a family, raise children—all the tangible things that become living proof of that love. Hoping that this feeling will continue for the rest of our lives, we feel like we are in heaven. We feel we are unbeatable and that together nothing can stop us.

I know this firsthand, because it is the feeling I had shortly after I married my wife Pia and moved to the United States from our native Italy. I didn't dwell on the fact that I was leaving my family, my country, my native language, and everything I had built in my life so far. That was baggage I wasn't going to carry. But, in reality, when the two of us traveled across the world to create our new life together, I carried in my heart the memories of the life I had created thus far.

Soon after we arrived in this country, I found myself studying for the medical boards. First, I had to obtain a license to practice medicine here in the United States. Then I had to repeat my entire medical residency in order to retrain and reestablish my career here. But, despite the tremendous hurdles I would have to endure just to practice what I had already been doing in Italy (I was a medical professor at the university there when I left), it didn't matter, because I was in love.

It didn't matter because I had made the choice to follow a new path with my wife. Instead of feeling drained by the enormity of it all, I was bursting with energy. All my feelings of self-doubt or criticism just disappeared, because I was filled with love. Nothing could stop me. This is how it is for those who fall in love. Their boundaries are limitless. When you are filled with love you move forward, you create, you are filled with enthusiasm. I have been like this since I arrived in this country, for thirty-four years.

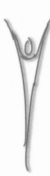

You have within yourself a wonderful power that only you can direct, the power of love. Love is at the core of your health, your happiness, and your life. But in order to give love, you must come to love and accept yourself, so it is of primary importance to listen and communicate with your inner voice, to be in tune with your spiritual heart.

Even now, when I wake up and realize I am across the globe from Italy, my homeland, I am excited and exhilarated about the things I still have to learn: new vocabulary, places to discover, people I have yet to meet. Love is a spark that animates everything in my life. It is the magic force that propels me.

So where does love come from? From what source does it spring forth?

The answer is simple: Our heart.

The will inspired by love is of an infinite magnitude. It springs forth from a never-ending well. The more one is fed by this source of love, the more love we are able to generate. It is a self-generating cycle and it starts in our hearts. The problem is that sometimes people or outside events obscure the immense propensity we have within ourselves to love, and we get hung up, or pushed down, or held back. The best way to improve your health is to have more love in your life. Health comes from a happy heart and a happy heart is one filled with love.

Love is always there waiting for us to tap into its source inside us. There will never be a moment in our lives when an act of love does not touch us deeply. It is like an immense, irresistible force. As I describe for you these experiences from my past, I am re-experiencing that strong feeling inside myself. I feel again how I felt when I came to this country, how Pia and I were driven by love and hoped that our dream would be fulfilled in our new home here.

THE POWER OF SELF-LOVE

We all have this wonderful force within our hearts, and it makes us unstoppable. There is no end to it. Knowing this, believing this, I wonder, why not use this powerful force to benefit us? Why do some people tap into it, and others not? Why don't we all catch on? Pondering this, I decided to create a simple exercise that will help you realize more self-love.

Exercise

To begin, close your eyes and visualize a time in your life when you were in love. Remember when you met the person who touched your heart so deeply you could not let go of this feeling. You felt like this person would be your soul mate, your companion for life. As long as you were alive, you wanted this person to be with you in love. How did that feel? How does that feel?

Do you see from this exercise how all the loving thoughts inside you come from your heart? Indeed, your heart is a source of love. Within your heart you store the memories and experiences of love you have received throughout your life.

Now, immerse yourself in the source and feeling of that love that has embraced you all your life. Imagine that you are weightless, unbound; you are riding on the waves of this love that magically carries you, as if free floating and suspended from the sky. You feel totally free. Relax. Remember your eyes radiant, a beautiful smile spreading across your face. You are pulled forward by an irresistible force that is the force of love. The force has never left you. Bring it to life.

This force has the power of sunlight. It is warm, comforting, rejuvenating, and enthusiastic. It fills you with energy, with a zest for life and creativity. Imagine that this golden light is flooding your head, flowing gently like a river to your face and neck, to your arms, and to your forearms and fingers, to your chest, to your abdomen and back, to your pelvic area, and to your thighs, down through your legs to your feet and toes. Every cell in your body is bathed in light. You are totally immersed in this ocean of love.

Always remember this great power of love within you. You can direct this power to love to yourself or others. Make it a daily experience. Fill yourself with this knowledge of love and the sense that you are peaceful, fulfilled, and happy.

These are not special feelings or unique experiences of love that should be felt only a few days of the year, such as the holidays or when you are on vacation. Let this feeling of love permeate your mind, body and soul. Every time you choose this experience, you will feel rejuvenated and renewed.

SHARING MY OWN STRUGGLE

Self-love has always been a critical issue in my own life. I, too, had to struggle with this. For most of us, self-love starts at the very beginning and is learned through our first relationships, with our parents. I know in my mind that my parents loved me immensely. I will be forever grateful for their dedication to us, but I recall feeling deprived because I wasn't told I was loved. I don't remember, for example, my father ever holding me.

Once, I asked my mother if my father loved me. She laughed: "Of course, he loved you so much." I realized this as an adult, when I was living far from our hometown in Sardinia. He came to visit me and we spent an entire day together, eating lunch, talking, and enjoying each other's company. When it was time for him to leave, he gave me a long, strong hug, got on the train, then a boat and traveled the long distance home. I didn't realize then that one day he would no longer be around.

When I moved to the United States, I made an annual journey back to visit my entire family, keeping a promise I had made when I left. But one year, I received a phone call that my father was very ill. I flew back to Sardinia and found him lying in a hospital bed, pale and weak, but very happy to see me. He asked me: "Bruno, are you happy in the States?" I said: "Yes," and he said: "That's all I want to know." I spent ten days with him; I gave him my blood for a transfusion and then I flew back to Chicago.

About a week later, I received a second phone call. My father had died. My brother Nello told me that when he was dying he cried out: "Bruno, Bruno, America." My brother said to my father: "Here is Bruno, here is Bruno," and put his hand under my father's hand. Because my brother did that, my father died peacefully. I will always be grateful.

Why do I tell you this now, when I am writing about self-love? It is because I realize now how important parents and authority figures are in inspiring self-love and self-trust. At an early age, when we don't know who we are, we see ourselves through the eyes of the people who love us. This is why I recall how I learned about love; I realize it was there for me through my parents. I didn't see it then, unfortunately, but I realize it now.

In fact, I started carrying my father's picture in my briefcase when I would go to the hospital to see patients. I wanted to visualize my father and see him at these times when I needed him. One day I asked my spiritual teacher about this and he looked at me and said: "Bruno, are you trying to get your father's love back?" I was quite surprised at this question, because it was so direct. I answered: "Yes." And he looked into my eyes even more intently and said: "You won't get it." It was a cruel reality.

I'M SURE THAT for you, too, there is a moment in life when you realize you have to let go of some painful memories of the past, memories of people you loved who are no longer with you. At this point, you must begin to parent yourself, to be a loving parent to yourself. I was one of five children. We all attended the university on limited family funds. My father had to work more than one job to do this for us, but he never once complained to me about anything. He silently did his work and dedicated his life to us.

My mother also is a strong reminder to me of this lesson. I remember her always working, working to prepare meals, to take care of the house. She was a perfectionist, but all this busyness left little time to pay attention to us, her children. I sometimes felt lonely and abandoned and learned that to get love and attention I had to perform, to do well.

Self-love was a struggle for me from early on. I was lucky though, in that my mother's sister, my Aunt Amelia, became an early teacher of love for me. I remember her always being happy, singing. She had a lot to handle in her life. She lived with my grandmother and her brother, who was an alcoholic and no good at taking care of the home. My aunt had to run the family manufacturing business.

I had a defining moment in my life. I was about six and had gone to the barber to get my hair cut. He cut my long hair off. When I went home, my mother opened the door, then quickly closed it saying: "You are not my son." I was devastated. I went to my aunt's house. When she opened the door, she laughed, hugged me, and I felt safe with her.

Another experience that taught me about love was when I was being tutored by a teacher at his house and he handed me a poem called "The Rock." It was about facing difficulty in life. I remember crying as he read the poem to me. I was fourteen years old. That moment changed my life. I learned to endure despite all adversity. It was up to me to become what I could and so I studied hard and never stopped trying from that moment on. I learned that love comes from the inside, that even if I felt that people around me didn't love me enough, it was up to me to love myself.

This journey has been a lifelong struggle for me.

My ticket to success was studying hard. It helped me surmount the family feuds at home, to receive top grades at the university, to leave my homeland and travel to the United States—to start over, begin a family and take up a new career.

THE TURNING POINT

A nagging inadequacy always haunted me. Despite all I was achieving, I never felt good enough, successful enough. I did research. I created a laser laboratory and traveled with this new technology, Then one day, I woke up and realized I was running away from myself, from my family. I was on the treadmill of success, traveling to Japan and Australia, working harder and harder to receive professional rewards.

I decided it was time to stop. I began to search for personal and spiritual growth. I was lucky to find a wonderful spiritual teacher in Carleton Whitehead. He helped me to discover myself, to love myself for who I was and not what I had accomplished. It was a breakthrough moment in my life, a turning point.

I learned that I was more than a physician, father, and teacher. I was a sensitive human being that had decided to dedicate his life to helping others. In fact, my main reason for being a physician was to prolong and save lives.

This led me to open a new office and to create a special backroom where my patients and their families could gather. There, I started giving talks about the prevention of heart disease. I began to share my own personal struggle and discovered the beauty of the patient/physician relationship. For the first time, I was dropping my mask with my patients as we all opened our hearts to a new way of healing. We began to share love through our stories and experiences. I learned by working and talking with them, that there was a font of self-love inside myself I didn't realize was there.

At the same time, I began to educate myself about holistic medicine. I attended talks by some of the leaders in this field, including Elisabeth Kübler-Ross, who was a model of love for dying people. I traveled to Sausalito, California, to see Gerald Jampolsky, who had dedicated his life to helping terminally ill children. I spent time training with him at his center, The Center for Attitudinal Healing. Children and their families would gather there to find healing in the experience of death or recovery.

Bernie Siegel became another role model for me. I was impressed by his work with cancer victims and the love and support that he gave to his patients, shifting their perception from illness to new possibility. Deepak Chopra showed me the path to self-love. He is a spiritual teacher for me. I learned from him about Ayurvedic medicine, the practice of meditation and the immense joy that is within when you silence the outside voices and get in touch with your spirit.

UNCONDITIONAL SELF-LOVE

It is truly difficult to find someone who doesn't want to be loved. Love is at the core of our health, our happiness, and our life. Without love, without self-love especially, there is no energy, no spiritual flame that lights our lives.

But love is unconditional. The more love we give, the more we will be loved in return. If we want to love, we must first give love. Simple. The same goes for respect, for judgment. It all applies to the biblical passage: "Do unto others what you want to be done to you." To give is to receive.

Sometimes, and too often, we forget these fundamental principles of life. We're overwhelmed by the pressures of our daily lives and forget to love without expectation. This is why it is so important to feed our spiritual heart with love, to keep this flame burning, and to nurture ourselves with compassion and patience.

Self-Acceptance

How do you look at your heart?

Through my years of experience I have found it to be really true that what we perceive as reality isn't always the true reality. Especially when it comes to our hearts. We often use metaphors to describe our heart feelings. For example, we say, "My heart is scarred." Or, "I have a big heart." "My heart is weak."

These metaphors can change our perception immediately. Cardiac patients, for example, are forced by their illness to look at their hearts. But sometimes their image is what other people create for them. By changing this image, we can change our behavior and attitude toward life. If we say, for example, "My heart is strong and can compensate for itself," it opens the door to healing. It allows us to see hope and new possibilities for the future.

Here is a powerful metaphor I would like you to try: "I give a hand to my heart in the walk of life." If you feel that your heart is wounded, you can heal it. You have the ability to heal yourself. Use it. As I was writing this, I found a small card on my desk that reads: "My faith deepens with each passing day. I trust in the goodness of life to sustain me and I give thanks to the grace of God that strengthens me now. God's faith is mine now."

Begin today. Start using powerful and creative new metaphors, full of possibilities. Rise above negative messages and empower yourself with the possibility of changing them. Become your own best friend.

TRANSFORMING PAIN INTO LOVE

Let me illustrate what it means to transform pain into love with some examples. Janet is a university professor who underwent several operations on her shoulder because of pain. The operations were not successful and she was incapacitated. Later, she developed a heart condition that required two angioplasties. Still, she continued her life as a teacher and became an artist. She projected her pain into love and produced paintings that are renowned.

Mary is a patient in her late thirties who I met while making hospital rounds. When I entered the room I saw her in bed resting. She had an arm amputated and was nearly blind because of diabetes, and she was on dialysis. When I asked her how she felt, she looked at me and said, "I am blessed. I am blessed." She was able to look beyond the body to the spiritual domain.

Kathryn is a ninety-year-old, frail woman who had open-heart surgery and was suffering from heart failure and diabetes. She lives alone in a mobile home and is surrounded by her dog Alexis and several cats. She has a zest for life. Having these animals with her and being awakened by them every day is enlivening for her. She would deprive herself of food to make sure her "children" are okay. When she was hospitalized she had one worry: Alexis and her cats? "Would you like to see pictures? The latest cat (Bam-Bam) has a black tail and these little blue eyes," she said smiling.

TELL YOUR OWN STORY

It is very important to write what you believe about your spiritual heart: This way, you can see the words; they are like feedback—you can relate to them. They also reveal where you are right now, at this time. It is a point of reference for the future. In addition, writing involves introspection and introspection is a necessary process for spiritual growth. I remember one author saying that not writing is like wanting to see yourself in a mirror without a mirror. When you write, in essence, the words are like a mirror. They mirror your spirit.

Exercise

Let your heart talk. Open your heart to yourself. The spirit within will uncover itself and open your eyes to the spiritual treasures within yourself. Be the person that your soul wants to be. Write your words so they can mirror your creative spirit. Give life to your infinite potential and let the voice of your spiritual heart be heard.

AN INNER DIALOGUE—WHO AM I?

The thrust of the above exercise is to help you get in touch with your spiritual heart, to learn to listen and communicate with your inner voice. You are not your work. You are not your reputation. You are not finished becoming you. And you can be in touch with your inner spirit.

Meditation

A voice within tells me,
I am your spirit.
God created me.
I am eternal.
I am not your work.
I am not your actions.
I am.
I always will be.
I am the voice of God.
In me you find what you seek.
You will always find me.
I am the essence of you.
And I love.
I always love you.
Fear not.
Find rest.
Stop searching.
In me is all you need.
Abandon yourself to the spirit within.
Let it be your guide,
*   your light in the path of life.*
Your spiritual self is the voice of God
*   whispering with infinite love.*
I am near you.
I lead you.
I keep you safe.

CHAPTER SIX

Your Spiritual Support System

"When my heart was quivering,
I remained calm and called my support group."
—A PATIENT

SUPPORT GROUPS

What is a cardiac support group? It is a group of like-minded people, with similar experiences, who meet periodically and share of themselves. In such a group no one person assumes the authority to direct the conversation and say, "This is what you should do!" They all realize that being open and sharing from the heart is fundamental for living a full life and for healing.

The key point is a paradigm shift from the wounded ego of the heart patients to the freedom of the spiritual domain. This happened to the exceptional heart patients I identified in my support group. I would like to share two of their stories. The first one is Jennifer's story.

THE COURAGE TO TAKE ACTION

Jennifer: "I was driving in the rain and I got halfway to work when I felt this pain start. The pain was right in the middle of my chest. It started getting worse and worse. I tried belching and thought, *This is not normal.* I started racing my car so I could get to a light where someone could find me. I knew I was in trouble.

"I pulled over and called 911. That was about ten minutes. They were there in less than five minutes. They came and gave me two nitros, one at a time. Nothing was happening. My blood pressure was high. The bottom number was 100. I remember that. I started getting the pain. It was moving toward the back, and they gave me morphine and aspirin. When they gave me the morphine, that calmed the pain. Then I was on my way to the emergency room.

"I got nauseated, but they said it was only because of the morphine. It left me right away. What went through my mind? *I'd better get help real fast!* I knew something was not normal.

"A couple of weeks before the episode I was doing a lot of heavy lifting. I moved a bookcase, and I was moving books. The cat jumped up on the highboy and fell, or jumped, down the back. The two sides are flush to the wall. He went down there and was meowing and meowing and making these noises, jumping

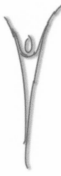

There are a variety of spiritual support systems available to you. Having the support of friends and loved ones is a fundamental part of our happiness. You may also wish to find help from others in learning the language of your spiritual heart. One thing you will learn for sure is that you will become your own best friend by making the effort.

and trying to get out. But he couldn't. I thought, *I have to get him out of there.* So I started pushing against the dresser to try to move it. Somehow, I don't know how, I found the strength. Like they say, you find it. I moved the cabinet far enough away even though it was full of stuff.

"The cat got out and was fine, but he scared me. I was worried. How was I going to get him out of there? I never experienced chest pains before that."

Dr. Cortis: "What went through your mind when they told you that you needed to do the balloon?"

Jennifer: "I got real scared because I heard you can stroke and then you have to have open-heart surgery. I didn't know I was having a heart attack at the time. I assumed I was. No one came out and told me that. I didn't want to

97

have this procedure done, not for a minute. Then I thought, *What am I, crazy? It is either that or I could have a stroke.* I signed up for it."

Dr. Cortis: "What did you feel when the balloon was inflated?"

Jennifer: "Nothing. I was out like a light. They had me in twilight sleep, but I was really more sleeping than anything else. I could see things as I woke up. I heard the doctor say I was sleeping."

Dr. Cortis: "When it all went well, how did you feel?"

Jennifer: "I got the shakes real bad. Then I felt really good. I thought, *Why the heck with all I am doing should I have this?* Now I think this is genetic. In May, as you know, the levels were terrific. My cholesterol was down, the triglycerides, the HDL were all good. I think that maybe this plaque had started before I did this alternative thing. What are you going to do?"

Dr. Cortis: "Did you start talking to your heart? Did you try to talk or were you just scared?"

Jennifer: "I was scared. I did get help. I don't know how long it will last. I have changed my perspective on things."

Dr. Cortis: "In what way?"

Jennifer: "Knowing how fast I could die, and then having another chance to be here."

THE SECOND STORY is equally dramatic. We are familiar with parental love: It is deep. It is powerful. It is life-changing. Pat was an only daughter and her parents focused all their care and devotion on her. Having seen her father Frank suffer from heart problems, Pat was studying to be a nurse. Her love could be channeled toward helping others. All was going well, until one day when Pat was on vacation.

Frank had been waiting for two years for a donor when a phone call informed him that Pat had been involved in a fatal car accident. Moments later a second call came, this time from the organ transplant coordinator: "Would you accept your daughter's heart?" Pat's love for her dad had inspired her to sign her license to be an organ donor. Her ultimate generosity directed that her body organs be preserved to help others live.

"How difficult it is to decide when you are the father of the donor and the recipient at the same time," Frank told me. Overcoming strong emotions, and guided by his loving wife, Frank found the strength to accept. To my knowledge, this is the only case of a transplant recipient having this experience. "She died so I could live," he said to me. "Every beat of her heart is a gift of life to me."

Frank is now dedicating his life to promoting organ donation so that other lives may continue living.

WORDS OF WISDOM FROM MY CARDIAC SUPPORT GROUP

Dr. Cortis: "My plan is to disclose the positive elements that promote your health. My objective is to empower you with knowledge in terms that you can understand. As we open our heart, we discover ourselves."

Margaret: "I would like to see my hospital develop a support group, because I thought the exercise program was very good, but people would all gather in the little tiny locker rooms and talk about everything with each other. We all had these experiences we needed to share and we don't think the program director ever really did talk to us honestly. When they got us together it was always for lectures. There was no discussion. Everything they showed us suggested that if a man had a heart attack, I, the woman, had to be a really good helper, and half the group was women.

"Nobody said anything about the women, so there was this funny discrepancy. So I told my doctor that I thought we should have a support group like Dr. Ornish described in his book *Dr. Dean Ornish's Program for Reversing Heart Disease* (Random House, 1990), so that some of us could work on those other issues. He said, 'What for?' I said, "For stress and everything.' He said, 'Well, I don't think so. A lot of people will be in more stress sitting in a group than if they didn't go to one. You know how people feel. Telling a group something and being candid is very hard for a lot of people.' So he didn't think there was any particular virtue in that. A very nice guy, but not interested in any of this. . . ."

Elizabeth: "I would like to say that my internist doesn't know I'm here this evening."

William: "Well, we will keep it a secret."

Elizabeth: "After my mastectomies I had no interest in going to a support group for breast cancer because I told myself I was no longer a cancer patient. The cancer was gone. I believe in positive thinking. In this I see that it is an on-going thing and that we need support because it is a total life change—every day of your life."

Marshall: "I've noticed changes, even since you came in here. When you first came in you were very quiet. (Laughter) I bet you thought you were going to just sit back and let us do all the work. (Lots of laughter)"

Elizabeth: "I don't know what happened. I brought a notebook and a pen and I was going to jot down all these ideas. I was all set very method-ically to take all these notes and find out all the different views. I haven't taken a single note, but I have learned a lot. Thank you. . . ."

James: "If you are interested in finding out about foods, I think all of us here would be more than happy to share what we know. Food is a very big thing. I guess it sounds like we are always talking about it. Going out to restaurants, you have to call and talk to them and ask for their help. Sometimes they are very nice. The better the restaurant, the more they will help. That is what we found out anyway."

Marshall: "That's right. I found that whenever I would call ahead to a restaurant, I would even ask to talk to the chef. Sometimes you can get to them. If he is the kind of Italian chef who can't cook without olive oil, he will be honest with you and then I won't go there. I talk to every restaurant the same way. . . ."

Dr. Cortis: "I love it that patients will talk to people about their own experiences. They are the most powerful teachers. Who better than a person with an experience to teach about it. We physicians are ineffective in touching people's hearts. To me, I feel patients are able to do that much more quickly."

Margaret: "My husband and I have a wonderful life and two wonderful children. I am one of those persons with a preexisting condition and if I have stress in my life it is because of the insurance companies who don't want to insure me. My father died when he was fifty of a massive coronary and my mother had high triglycerides and high cholesterol. So I knew I had a history of this. I had a stress test in my doctor's office and the doctor said it was not normal. This was just before the holidays and I said I don't want my kids remembering me dying around the holidays. I went to another doctor to see if the results were the same, and they were.

"Then I knew I had to do this and went into the hospital and made an appointment. They found I was 100 percent blocked on one side and 90 percent blocked on the other, so they went in and did the angioplasty. I asked the doctor while I was on the table how open he got the arteries, because you're awake and watching your heart on the two monitors. He said 100 percent. And, you know, it's painful because they have the balloon open and the blood shut off to your heart, and it's then they decrease it.

"Then I go right away into cardiac rehab for I don't know how many sessions, and after that I'm supposed to stay on some kind of exercise. So we have a really good treadmill, but it gave me bone spurs, or I should say it allowed me to have bone spurs, so I couldn't work out on the treadmill. So I said, "Well, Lord, keep watching all these things I want to do." Then I heard of this thing called chelation therapy from four different sources so I knew it was of the Lord, and what I was to do.

"I came here to you because I wanted to know if I had any blockage and I didn't want to have another angiogram. So we did a thallium test and found out it was normal, praise the Lord. Today I was on the cross-country trainer for thirty-five minutes. Now we're going totally fat-free in our house, and eating more vegetables and salads. . . ."

Tom:
(Margaret's husband)

"She is right basically about the two things I would say this helps us for. One of the biggest problems we all have is stress because we live a very fast lifestyle and it causes a lot of problems. My cholesterol was up too and what we are trying to do now is eat right and exercise. The best thing that happened to her I think was the chelation. She was able to cut her medication down dramatically and the chelation has given her a lot more energy. She's got a lot more energy than I have. We will do anything that we try together and having something like this where people can talk about it is really key, because most of us fall by the wayside. . . ."

Marshall:

"My wife and I walk almost every evening when we can. Tonight we can't, so when I get home I will go on my treadmill. But generally we try to walk every evening, not a fast walk so that both of us feel exhausted, but a nice and easy walk. You notice the neighbor you never talked to, watch the kids playing in the street, see how people decorate their houses and yards. This is how I relax now, noticing things."

Alex: "My wife and I exercise religiously, not vigor-ously. Like the doctor said, you don't have to go out there and kill yourself. It has done wonders for her because she has her figure back that she had twenty years ago, and she lost twenty-six pounds. I've lost fifteen. And even the kids—we have a twenty-one-year-old and a sixteen-year-old—are now becoming aware of the stuff they are consuming and exercising more."

Dr. Cortis: "Let me share an experience I had. I was in California and I went to a restaurant. I went to the washroom and there was a mirror in front and one behind me. The mirror behind me showed my partially bald head. I said to myself, I can choose to look in the mirror in front of me which shows my hair or I can look at the back of my head in the mirror behind, which I don't much like. We have the power to choose which part of ourselves we like to love. This all has nothing to do with self-love. Self-love is self-acceptance, and you accept all of yourself. Our body is just the appearance; we have so much more beauty inside that just our body. Don't stop at the weight. Look inside yourself to know better who you are, what can be your contribution to the world. These are your most beautiful attributes. . . ."

James: "I was thinking about what you said about loving the parts of your body. I was at Dean

Ornish's program and a woman there taught us that we had to love our entire body, and that if you do you can then be aware of everything that is in your body that is good and bad. If you love it you can release it. But until you learn to love your whole body you can't release the plaque or the things in your body you want to get rid of. I was amazed when I first heard that. How can you love the plaque in your body? But, the way she explained it, it is part of your body and you accept it; and because it is part of your body you love it. Then you can release it."

Dr. Cortis: "Keep sharing of yourself. The trend in medicine these days is that mind and body are one. There are many studies showing that the brain produces substances that send messages to the body, but in turn the cells of the body produce the same substances that go to the brain. So the body is a network of information."

James: "It was six months ago that I had an angioplasty and it's a strange thing but I've watched myself get better along the way and build more confidence. I think it has a lot to do with the many things the people were talking about here this evening in terms of just treating myself better, taking care of myself physically, putting better things into my body. Trying to change old habits that are hard to change. It is unfortunate that the part of your body that needs to heal is the part that usually breaks down. In my case it is the heart.

"I've had to open my heart up in lots of ways to share things and be with people and do things differently and to make an effort to reach out and connect with people and to share things. I find myself getting better, stronger, just taking more time to enjoy things and not to be so rushed. I do the meditation in the morning and it helps me immensely in my day. I make an effort to be pleasant to people more, to listen more, and not flap my mouth so much. Everyday is something new; something different comes along. And I'm starting to enjoy it—I wish I could have done it earlier, but I'm doing."

Secrets of Achieving Longevity

In the practice of medicine I have interviewed a number of people in their nineties who were enjoying a normal life. What were their secrets? Here are some common traits:

- Ignoring their calendar age, but focusing on the vital energy they still enjoyed. How old they were was irrelevant. How young they felt was the issue.
- Moderating physical activity, but being active on a regular basis. They chose the type of exercise they liked the most—swimming, walking, or whatever. I am reminded of a Chinese proverb that says: "Don't worry about walking slowly, worry about not stopping."

- Eating a mixed diet. They ate a little of everything. When I questioned them about a specific regimen, one answered: "Why live like a sick person to die healthy?"
- Enjoying an active community life with friends and families.
- Keeping a good sense of humor. One woman came to my office with her X-rays and said: "Keep them here. They only hold them at the hospital for ten years." Another ninety-two-year-old confessed to me jokingly: "If I knew that I would have lived this long, I would have taken better care of myself."
- Maintaining a spiritual optimism and looking at the universe as a loving place.
- Holding on to a sense of purpose. Their life was full of meaning and their smile inspiring.

Samuel Ullman wrote these words about aging: "Youth is not a time of life. It is a state of mind. People grow older by deserting ideas. Years wrinkle the skin, but to give up enthusiasm wrinkles the soul."

And Voltaire said: "Those who do not appreciate what is unique about old age will only appreciate its loss."

HEART INVENTORY

Having friends and their support is a fundamental part of our happiness. We identify with them and they nourish us with affection and love. But it is equally important to be your own best friend. In your own heart you can find the spiritual help that makes us all be one.

Exercise

Take a good look at your heart. Stand back and imagine that you are a silent observer. What is the temperature of your heart? Is it warm, or is it cold? How close or how distant do you feel? What is your heart color? Is it a vibrant red? What is your heart's passion? What is the spiritual spark that enlivens your heart?

The Language of the Heart

Learning the language of the heart is not something that just happens all of a sudden. You need to give yourself the time and the place and the incentive to speak to your heart, to pay attention to your own inner voice. But you can be your own best ally by making the effort.

Meditation

Be attuned to the language of the heart.
It is the language of love.
God gave us the gift of life
*   and he put the seed of love in our heart.*
So think of the people you love
*   and who love you.*
Create a moment of spiritual union
*   thinking of them,*
*   wishing them well.*
Embrace them with love
*   and accept their attention.*

*This life is an opportunity for you
    to make visible the imprint of God
    in our lives.
Do not postpone it.
Do not ignore it.
Take advantage of the moment.
The time is now.
Let your heart find the words
    that evoke loving kindness
    and compassion
Be an ambassador of love.*

CHAPTER SEVEN

A Spiritual Home Within Your Heart

*"In the middle of this road we call our life,
I found myself in a dark wood
with no clear path through."*
—DANTE ALIGHIERI

SPRING CLEANING

When we talk about spring cleaning, of course, we are thinking of cleaning our house or the garage and setting everything in order. We never consider doing a spring cleaning of the negative emotions we carry in our heart, the bad memories we hold on to. "Is this important or relevant?" you may ask. Yes, and especially so because the way we feel from moment to moment, the way we behave, the actions we take are all conditioned to how we feel inside.

Feelings come from the heart: feelings of loneliness, feelings of low self-worth, feelings of sadness and worry.

Do you ever realize how important they are?

Honestly, it is critical that we consider carrying out a spring cleaning of our heart.

Let us start with childhood memories. There are phrases we repeat to ourselves that we heard as children. "Children are to be seen and not heard." "Will you stop that." Personally, I remember emotional isolation more than anything else. There were issues I could not discuss with anybody. I carried them within myself for decades. I was fearful of not helping other people. Appearances had to be perfect according to my parents. It was a lot pressure. I used to live in a small province of Italy and everybody knew about everybody else.

Then I graduated at the university and moved to Turin to study cardiology. In that environment I learned another lesson, and that was never to show your feelings. Always put up a good front.

I was in the midst of my own personal spring cleaning before I realized that what I intended to do was to go to a deeper level. I would like to open my heart and share one event that happened during my adolescent years. I have never shared the memory of it with strangers. I was maybe twelve or thirteen years old. I was innocent, beginning life almost, when the bus driver took my friend and myself to a bus and molested us. It only happened once and I was not aware of any real consequences. I went home. I have no other memories of it. My life continued. I was at that time in a little town in the mountains because there was a war going on. The military district that my father directed was moved from the city that was bombarded heavily, to a small town in the mountains where we all were safe. I continued to go to school and life was joyful.

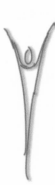

A re you aware of the feelings you are carrying in your heart? You may need to look inside your spiritual heart, discover and communicate with your inner child, perform a "spring cleaning" of unresolved emotions, and lighten the load of sadness you carry within. If you can fully accept, respect, and appreciate yourself, you can make peace with yourself.

The years went by and I cannot say at which exact moment things changed, but all of a sudden I experienced a sense of guilt, a sense of shame, a sense of violation. I did not know exactly what it was, but I was deeply ashamed of myself. I couldn't say anything about these feelings to anybody. It was the time of my life when I began to be aware of girls. In that small town where I was living that was also a secret. Nobody in my family knew it.

I still carried the memory. I did not say anything to anybody for many years, not even in confession, which seemed at the time for me to be a sacrilege.

One day, twenty years later, I shared the experience with my brother. We did not make anything of it. It was inconsequential. I felt the need to tell somebody, to unburden myself. I've never said anything to anyone else since.

Now I am once more opening my heart to myself. I realize how much pain and suffering that experience caused me in my life. I realize now more than ever what I mean by spring cleaning. It is exactly what I am doing, sharing the most painful experience in my life with humility, with serenity, without hate. I invite you to do the same with painful experiences.

IT WAS ACTUALLY wintertime when I first wrote down the above reflection. I was in church and I was observing the trees outside. All I could see were the naked branches. This is how we know the trees in the winter. The leaves that once filled out the branches are no longer there. They have fallen. The tree is naked.

This image became for me like an internal symbol of spring cleaning. Shake the things from your heart that should fall and be collected. We all need to recognize the uselessness of continuing to suffer, of wasting our emotional and spiritual energy with unresolved negative memories of the past.

Spring cleaning is such a healthy thing to do. And it's just the beginning; there is never an end. All our life we have to continue our spring cleaning. I don't think I ever met anybody who had completed the job.

Open your heart to yourself. Be truthful. Clear your path to God. When we are ashamed of ourselves we lose our naturalness and our spontaneity. We all like to assume a mask of perfection, and aura of invincibility. In truth, we cannot. The spiritual heart is where the spring cleaning starts and, as I say to myself, now's the time to start. I invite you to unburden yourself, and regain your emotional freedom. In the eyes of God you are invaluable.

Eventually, I shared the above experience with my wife and my son. This was also liberating, but it took me many years just to get to the point where I could do so. I wonder how many of us have still not done any spring cleaning.

What Do You Carry In Your Heart?

Here's an exercise to help get you started with your spring cleaning:

Exercise

Sit down in a comfortable place. Close your eyes and let go of people and circumstances. Find peace. Then look to your heart and identify the most painful experience you have ever had, the one whose memory was not to be shared with anybody. Think of that one thing that has had you convinced that if people knew about it you would lose their love. Examine your spiritual heart and release yourself from the grip of that constricting experience.

Write a Letter to a Lost Friend to Unburden Your Heart

Another way to work on your spring cleaning is to write a letter to someone you trust with your deepest concerns. This might be your spouse, your best friend, your mentor. It could be anyone. You can unburden your heart by sharing the weight of whatever you are experiencing. And remember, it's the exercise that is important, writing down the details of what has brought you pain. It may be a letter that you never send, but it gives you a format and a focus for expressing your concerns. I will give you an example here. I considered Dr. Whitehead my mentor, and this is what I would like to say to him.

Dear Carleton:

You know that I love you and that I have always loved you, and that I consider you my mentor, a person who accepted me without judgment, a person who evoked in me the best qualities of spontaneity and joy, laughter and humor.

You always inspired me to follow my spirit, and in doing so you gave me so many joys. My past conditioning molded me into a self-judging, self-pitying, and self-limiting person. My spirit was always grounded. You helped me. You gave me the idea of spiritual freedom. The idea that we are all born with the right to enjoy life, be happy, and fulfill our dreams and desires, and, most of all, the right to make mistakes, to change our mind, to be optimistic.

You also showed me how to be independent in my thinking and in my will, how to have a dignity of my own, and how to honor my spiritual self that is so beautiful, so sacred, and so neglected. My emotions are taking over. I feel a knot in my throat. I knew that there would be a moment of separation, but you always projected an image of strength, that a person with the power of mind can overcome an illness of the body. I entertained an image of your immortality, and you lived a very long, joyful life.

You always projected yourself toward enjoyment and fulfillment. In a sense, also, you were self-content; you were satisfied with what you had. As for myself, there is sometimes an element of self-sabotage, not being happy with what I have. Yet what I have is already so much. What am I going to do with it? I am always seeking more and missing what I have in the present.

This also I learned from you. Enjoy every moment in life. Enjoy life to the fullest. Be grateful. Not to envy was a lesson I learned from you, as was forgiving myself and loving myself. Most of the principles I wrote in my first book, *Heart and Soul,* came from your teaching. And for this, again, I am grateful.

You never asked for anything. You were simply happy that your spirit was infused in me and that because of your spirit I began seeking within myself the spiritual power we all have that only needs self-expression and fulfillment. Ultimately, you opened my heart to God. But the God you taught me was, as you said, a first-hand God, not a God up in the sky somewhere. Not a far-distant, judgmental, punishing God. You replaced that God with a loving God who is as close as my breath, a loving Father. And that freed me of a lot of my past conditioning and allowed me new joys in life.

You never feared death. I sensed that. You considered death as a transition. When you gave sermons for people who died, you used a poem from Kahlil Gibran, which pictured a boat that leaves a beach to move across the water to another place where people who loved that person are waiting. Death is just a transition from this world to another beautiful world. The reason why I am so deeply moved is because, as you will know, for me death has always been an issue, an issue of which I am still afraid.

I still have inner work to do. You called this work "clearing" and, in essence, this is what I am trying to achieve. This fear of death causes me a sense of anxiety, time pressure. I fear that I will not have enough time to accomplish the things I want to do. You remember, I told you that. I was afraid when my brother died because it happened so unexpectedly. At least, in my eyes he was only in his early seventies and we could have had so many years still together.

When I told you that I was afraid that something might happen to me before I can sing my song, you looked straight into my eyes and said: "You are terminal now." The bottom line was: Don't wait to discover that you are sick to run toward life. Live your life fully every day, now. Be grateful for what you have because it is not forever. Enjoy it! God wants you to enjoy it, you said. God is love, power, beauty, joy—and that is what you are. You said these words so many times

I salute you, Carleton. I thank you again for your lesson of love, for being a teacher of life and spirituality. The greatest one I have ever met. Thank you, Carleton. May you be in the arms of God.

Bruno

COMMUNICATING WITH YOUR INNER CHILD

I was raised in a family of six. I had a brother and two sisters who were older. I was the second to last child and I was literally isolated because my older brother and sisters would not play with me and my other sister was too young. So I found my main support in my friends. I specifically remember three of them: Carleno, the soccer champion; David, the pastry shop owner;

and Anthony, the lonely rich boy. Unfortunately, between the year I was eight and the year I was fourteen, they all died. Carleno died in a motorcycle accident; David died at home; and Anthony took his own life.

The key concept here is that the child within us is still alive and in need of love. We must keep in touch with this child so we can heal hurts that have been hidden and ignored for a long time. It is incredible how vivid the memories of my childhood and my father are.

I remember my father being busy most of the time. He was a colonel in the infantry and always wore tall leather boots and an expression of concern—an intimidating figure for me to address openly. He was too involved and I was too fearful, but I know now that he loved me to the point of calling my name when he was dying. Over the years I had become his preferred son. Maybe because we both had a gentle nature, humble, silent, and lonely. My mother had so much to do with her five children. She was always working, and again, I didn't perceive room for me to express myself at that age. The only opening for me was my Aunt Amelia who was unmarried and always in good spirits, the hardest working person I know of and always thinking of others—always concerned about how to give, never about receiving. I was told that she had a fiancé once but he went off to the war and died and she was never engaged again.

She showered her love on the family. She became our second mother. For me, she was like my only mother. The other person I could open my heart to was my confessor, Father Joseph, a Franciscan Friar. He was of middle height, stocky, rounded glasses with black frames, and a very friendly smile. He always wore brown sandals. Now and then I would receive a hug from him but many times I remember being scolded and warned about being a sinner and all the dangers of sin.

WHEN I STARTED at the university I put my heart into my studies. I was able to get excellent marks, maximum cum laude. I discovered that this was a way to be acknowledged, admired, and feel confident, so I stuck with it and studied harder and harder. Another reason was that I wanted to save money for the family and by getting good marks I could avoid paying tuition. In addition to that, a small scholarship was provided for needy students like me, "students who were deserving due to their grades and in need at the same time. That was the terminology. The Italian words were *Studenti Meritevoli Bisognosi.*

The six years of university flew by. Before I knew it I was a physician and had moved out of the house. Emotionally I was unprepared, although I had acquired a large body of knowledge. Years of studying, getting my Ph.D., specializing and writing for medical journals, participating in professional meetings, coming to the States, getting married, having children, and creating a family—it all went so fast. Throughout all this time I lost all awareness of my inner child. I only got in touch with him again when I took a course on self-development and learned about the inner child of the past. Then I had a healing experience.

The major crime, if I could imagine it as such, was the sense of abandonment that I felt. I feel that I abandoned my parents and my family first by wanting to go to the northern part of Italy to study cardiology and then by immigrating to the United States. The need to do these things was far stronger within me than the need to remain on the island where I was born. I needed freedom for self-expression and in the small town where I grew up I felt overwhelmed by the social stratification and the inability to change it. The social structure was such that status was conferred upon an individual by birth. Whoever was high on the social scale was assured that position for life; everything was settled. I had neither influential parents nor financial means, so I was at a disadvantage.

The solution to all my problems was to leave my city and my family in search for what I wanted most, freedom to be me, freedom of self-expression. The other imaginary crime, I would say, was the guilt I felt because I left; because I didn't spend as much time with my parents as I should have (or could have); I felt guilty because my father died when I was in the States and I was not with him; and when my sister Leda died I felt guilty. I was in the States and didn't help her enough. We loved each other so much.

I remember my brother called me to tell me that she had died two days after having surgery. I felt overwhelmed, destroyed. I went back home from the office and put a few things into an empty suitcase and I flew all night long back to Sardinia. This time at the airport the experience was totally different. It was not summertime so there were only a few passengers there. Instead of hugs and kisses from the whole family, only three people came, my brother and his son and daughter. We hugged each other and then they took me straight to where my sister's coffin was waiting.

I found her lying in a metal coffin. Her eyes were closed. She was asleep forever. The image I carried of her was of a charming, sweet person smiling, welcoming me with a hug. This time she was immobile. Her hands were crossed. A rosary was in her hands. I felt the need to kiss her and hug her. I kissed her hands and brought them to my face as if she was caressing me. I kissed her feet. Then I put both arms around her and I lifted her up as if we were hugging each other. Her skin was cold. Her eyes were closed. I put her back down. My brother and his wife took me away.

The coffin had to be closed. We got into our cars and followed the hearse to church. This time the coffin was close to the altar and Mass was celebrated. Around her coffin was a black and golden band with her name and flowers all around. I met old friends that I had not seen for almost ten years. We were all saddened by the sudden disappearance of Leda.

CONNECTING WITH YOUR INNER CHILD

You will never regret reconnecting with your inner child, the source of your joy, laughter, spontaneity, and naturalness. Open your heart to him or her, and listen attentively.

Exercise

Imagine that you are seated in a comfortable chair, relaxed, with your eyes closed. Visualize yourself when you were four or five years old. Then visualize this child sitting on your lap. Imagine you are looking into his or her eyes and you are losing yourself in the depth of that innocent look. The child keeps looking at you and displays an unspoiled spontaneity, enthusiasm, and zest for life.

Imagine that you hug him (or her), that you embrace him, because this is the child's language. It is the language of love. Then listen to what this child has to say. Listening creates the bridge of communication where the child expresses his needs and the adult discovers what his own needs are. You have all these qualities within yourself, in the child that you were, in the adult that you are.

If you have difficulty doing this exercise, just find a picture of yourself at a very early age, three or four years old. Use a magnifying glass to look into the eyes in the picture. Put yourself in touch with that part of yourself that is the most genuine, the most sensitive, the most loving. You need that child's support to bring to memories to light, to reawaken feelings, to nurture your spirit.

REPLACING THE NEGATIVE WITH THE POSITIVE

We have always made the connection between the mind and the body in general, and the heart and emotions in particular. The Type A personality, for example, has been determined to be a predisposing factor for coronary disease. Additional studies have shown that what is detrimental is not so much being in a hurry as it is the presence of hostility: frequent outbursts of anger and aggressive behavior. When hostility is high, there is an increase in heart attacks and even death. Physicians and lawyers seem to be typically susceptible.

Intense emotions during catastrophic events affect our cardiovascular system. Some examples include the stresses caused by the war in Israel or the earthquake in Los Angeles. In both cases the number of cardiac events rose and then returned to normal a few days later.

Even occasions such as the Olympics demonstrate the correlation. There were eight heart attacks and two sudden deaths during the 1996 Olympics. Again, it was because of emotional stress. It has been noted that depression also increases the incidence of heart attacks. During periods of bereavement, especially the first three days, there is a significant increase in acute myocardial infarctions and sudden death.

Conversely, there are psychosomatic elements that are supportive of our body defense mechanism. I would say positive emotions, such as having personal support and love, even the love of animals. Just the presence of an animal at home increases the possibility of survival and reduces heart attack because of the link of love. The visits of a chaplain to hospital patients have shortened their hospital stay. Even the room where we are in the hospital has an effect. Where the view is only that of the parking lot the recovery rate may be less than when the exposure is different and we can see flowers blooming and hear the birds singing. The connection to our cardiovascular system is subtle, but we can no longer neglect this fundamental aspect of our being.

LIGHTENING THE LOAD OF SADNESS

One of our major burdens is when we load our heart with sadness. Sadness in its essence may include some guilt and deep inside the real reason for our guilt is our difficulty in forgiving ourselves or others. Why should we forgive? After all, we have been deeply hurt. Let's reconsider everything within our grasp and free ourselves of this emotional baggage.

Yes, we made mistakes. So what! Have you met anybody in your life who was perfect? The answer obviously is no. So we all make mistakes. The most important step is that we forgive ourselves, that we accept ourselves with our painful memories. In this act of acceptance we free ourselves of that load.

Forgiveness has been said to mean giving love to yourself and others. In reality, when we forgive ourselves and we forgive others this is an act of true love. We release the pain, the anger, and the resentment that we have been holding within ourselves.

Maybe I can give you an image. Imagine yourself carrying a weight on your back. The weight becomes heavier and heavier. You bend over from the weight, but you are not willing to let go. As you forgive, you let go of the weight; you are again able to walk upright; you regain the freedom to be.

Forgiveness is not only an act of love; it is an act of self-interest in that we decide to no longer hurt ourselves. The anger we keep inside is like an imaginary flame that is burning us as we hold it. Why shed more tears over a problem of the past that is gone forever. As we forgive, we heal ourselves and this is one of the ultimate goals of our life. Consider, also, that unforgiveness consumes vital energy. Wouldn't it be more meaningful to redirect this power to our self-healing? Imagine the person you want to forgive on a stage. That person is receiving applause from the audience. You join the people applauding and supporting that person. This act of love and support is in itself healing.

THE UNEXPRESSED HEART

One of the greatest joys in life is to live with authenticity, with your life actions and your soul aligned. Not expressing your heart desires, ignoring the inner voice, not seeking fulfillment can affect your heart and your life.

When I first met Carl, he was the medical director of a New York hospital. I liked him because of his interests in culture and philosophy and for his open-mindedness. I believe that his job, however, involved too much stress. One day, unexpectedly, he suffered a heart attack. It was a great surprise for everyone. He was hospitalized and I went to see him; his wife was also there. He recovered and gradually resumed his work as if nothing had happened. He kept his hospital job, in addition to his medical practice, which in my view again was way too stressful.

One day, he opened his heart to me and told me that, in truth, his real love was writing and public speaking, affecting others, teaching others. He said that he spoke to his heart and told himself that not doing anything was not living. So he declared, "I told my heart that I want to have a full life, and if it follows me, fine. If it doesn't, then we will both die together." These were his words. They are still alive in my mind because of the circumstances—Carl died. When they told me that he had died, it didn't seem real. I remembered that just a few days before when I saw him in the hospital he was laughing and teasing me because I had changed my hairstyle and he had said, "Boy, you look younger."

Carl has left this world. I was informed that he was found in the shower, the water running. There was no response. I can imagine the tragedy of discovering his body and I feel sad. Carl was only forty-seven.

THE WAY TO HAPPINESS

To listen to the spirit within, you must consciously choose to silence all other voices that are seeking your attention. These voices can be the voice of power, the voice of control, the voice of achievement. You must simply surrender to the voice of the spirit. The goal of this exercise is to find and talk to the spiritual part of yourself. The language of the spirit is the only language of real value. It is the voice that connects you to inspiration, to peace, to love and meaning. Connecting to this voice is the ultimate reality and it will help you discover your spiritual treasure.

It all starts with surrender, with the conscious decision to admit that real happiness is not found in the material world. Self-contentment lies within—within you. It is always available and waiting to be discovered by you.

Exercise

Inner peace is related primarily to self-acceptance, the capacity to say to yourself meaningfully, I accept, I respect, and I appreciate myself. Examine how comfortable you are with yourself, with who you are. Make peace with yourself!

LISTEN TO YOUR BODY

Your body is the vehicle that carries you through life. "Treat your body like a temple," says the Bible. Listen to your body's messages, and take action.

Meditation

My body has a gentle way of calling for attention.
   "Hey! Hey!" the body whispers.
And then a little louder,
   "Hey! Hey!" I'm talking to you.

And when I keep going the body says
  "Wham! I've got your attention now!"
I am ill again.
I didn't listen, again.
Is my body happy?
No!
My body knows that I'm heading to the doctor
  so I can get well quickly.
My body is asking for love and concern
  and all I can think of is antibiotics.
And still my body tries to communicate with me,
  establish a healing dialogue,
  like a friend.

I'm going to make peace with my body.
I need to give it some respect,
  some love.
Especially my heart.
I promise myself to listen
  to my heart's signals
  as messages from the soul.
They are meant to draw my attention
  toward a problem
  that needs loving care.
My heart is the center of life.
My health is the most precious gift I have.

CHAPTER EIGHT

Quiet Your Mind to Hear Your Heart

"The longest journey that you will make in your life is from your head to your heart."
—GARY ZUKAV (*THE HEART OF THE SOUL*)

FINDING SPIRITUAL TIME

We often hear the idea that inner peace is born of outer conditions. We say to ourselves, "Tonight, when I finish my work, I will have some peace." "When I complete these obligations, I will finally get some rest." "When I find companionship, I will experience tranquility."

How can we achieve serenity in a world that is in constant motion, when we are pressed by demands and expectations? The solution comes, as Carleton Whitehead says, when we have brought our thoughts, feelings, and actions into harmony with the innermost core of our being, the divine within. We experience peace when we stop looking for outer conditions that will rescue us and we rely only on our inner resources. The center of peace is within ourselves.

We are truly an individualization of God's Spirit. In the incredible inner space that is the spiritual heart, we experience moments of harmony and balance that are inherent to our nature. These moments I call "islands of peace." This is the peace that Jesus referred to by saying, "Peace I leave with you, my peace I give to you." It is the oneness with the universe that creates the peace we need.

As we live in this domain, we nurture our divine spirit and in turn are cherished by it. Here are some of the ways. We attune ourselves to his realm by being in touch with nature. Just looking at a tree, for example, one is conquered by its majesty and its stillness, by its full growth into many branches, outstretched like arms to embrace the universe, while its leaves constantly face the blue sky. To me the tree becomes a symbol of the unity of nature with God.

I have experienced beautiful moments of peace looking at the ocean early in the morning, where I could see as far as the horizon, where the sea and the sky unite. I felt the same peace in Colorado contemplating the beautiful snow-covered mountains standing like giants under the blue skies. I sense serenity looking into the innocent eyes of a child, eyes that are still clear and focus without fear. How wonderful it is to discover these moments of spiritual richness when we feel close to God.

People who are able to remain healthy and productive in the midst of a busy life are those who develop the ability to alternate intense periods of purposeful activity with periods of respite from all tasks, responsibilities, and worries. In a nutshell, healthy, productive people move back and forth between productive time and time to recharge themselves. You have the

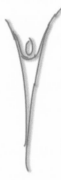

Your mind never stops going. Your world is in constant motion. You need to create "islands of peace" for yourself to help move back and forth between productive and recuperative time. You can do this by using affirmations and visualizations, by connecting with your spiritual heart through meditation, by awakening your consciousness and mastering your attentiveness.

ability to provide yourself with these islands of peace. They are the keys to gaining control of your life and unstressing yourself. So what can you do for yourself to achieve peace of mind? How can you interrupt the stresses and responsibilities of your daily routine and move into the inner space of your spiritual heart? How do you create balance in your life?

Exercise

Take a blank piece of paper and give yourself five minutes to brainstorm possible ways to create islands of peace in your life.

AFFIRMATIONS

To affirm means to make a statement of truth. Affirmations are positive statements that we repeat to ourselves about a situation or a specific problem we have in mind, and we do it either in a silent way or out loud.

131

Why do we need affirmations? What are the positive results we expect from them? Affirmations help us create the state of mind we wish to have. Affirmations provide positive energy, so repeat to yourself statements such as: "God is my partner." "I accept my spiritual nature." "I prosper from the harmony of life."

Positive affirmations have an uplifting effect and when repeated regularly, in essence, change our thinking and our feelings. Louise L. Hay, author of *You Can Heal Your Life* (Hay House, 1999), advises us to repeat these affirmations in front of a mirror. In so doing, we bring forth the same affirmation and if we experience any negative emotions, we can eliminate them. A critical component of affirmations is our faith that what we petition will happen. If we don't believe that we are worthy of receiving these gifts, our positive statements will lose their power.

THE FUNCTION OF FAITH

What is faith? Faith is a mental attitude. Faith is an approach to reality. Faith is the law of belief. Do I believe that this thing can be done? If so, then it can be done. The law of faith is like any other law in nature. When I plant a seed, I have faith that a plant will be generated. I have faith that the day will follow the night. In a sense, we live in a spiritual universe where everything is governed by law. It is the law of belief and connection.

Faith is the use of our spiritual power. We have faith when we become aware of it. What do I believe because of faith? I believe that the essence of the universe is spiritual. I believe that the Spirit of God is in everything and everywhere. I believe that

I am part of the spirit of God. As such, I am endowed with the same spiritual attributes. It is up to me to become aware of them and accept them.

When we say that faith can be acquired, it means that we can increase our awareness of faith. Faith can be practiced. We can practice the belief that all is well, that God protects us, that we are all brothers and sisters, that the essence of life is the spirit and that spirituality transcends the physical world.

VISUALIZATIONS

When we visualize something that we want, we visualize it in the present. Our brain experiences this mental picture as if it was something real and it becomes a part of our experience. Athletes often use visualization techniques. They see themselves practicing an exercise step by step in their mind. When they perform the action they have already run the same event many times in their mind. Golfers are taught to picture every shot. Divers visualize each dive before they step up onto the diving board.

If a patient has a heart problem, why not envision the heart as a powerful muscle that is full of energy and regains strength every day? When we practice visualization, we should use all our senses so that we make the experience as real as possible. Imagine a beautiful mountain in vivid color. Imagine the breeze caressing your face on the summer beach. Feel the warmth of the sun. Listen to the rustle of the leaves under a tree.

CONNECTING WITH YOUR HEART

According to Sogyal Rinpoche, "Meditation is not something you can do; it is something that happens spontaneously." He compares our mind to a candle flame that is unstable and flickering, constantly changing. Similarly our mind changes because of thoughts and emotions. The secret of meditation is to create an environment and let meditation happen. There is a correlation between the posture of the body and the attitude of the mind.

Exercise

To begin, be seated on the floor, or on a pillow. Visualize your posture—it should be like a mountain, expressing the core of your being. It is essential to keep your body straight, like an arrow. Cross your legs—they express life and death. Leave all your senses. All the light of your wisdom energy resides in your heart center, which is connected through wisdom channels to your eyes.

Keep your mouth slightly open and your hands covering your knees comfortably. One technique is to watch your breathing—breathing is the most fundamental expression of life. Focus about 25 percent of your attention on your breathing and 75 percent on just being quiet and relaxed. Each time you breathe out you let go and release your grasping. During meditation your mind is suspended in space . . . nowhere.

Rinpoche defines thoughts as the family of your mind. In the same way as the ocean rises and settles, we should allow our thoughts to rise and settle: "Thoughts are like the wind. They come and go. The secret is not to think about thoughts, but allow them to flow through the mind. When one thought is gone and the other has not come yet, there is a gap. In that silent gap is your spirit. With meditation we achieve the wisdom of egolessness."

During meditation you connect yourself with your heart essence, where God is present. What is important is the state of mind in which we find ourselves after meditation. It is peaceful, centered and calm.

Meditation is the road to enlightenment, a way to embody the transcendent while we are here. With meditation we become masters of our bliss and chemists of our joy.

Meditation helps the heart by causing physical changes, such as lowering the heart rate, blood pressure, oxygen consumption, and level of stress hormones. In addition, there are mental changes—we feel calm and serene; an emotional shield protects us and we experience an increased sense of control; time moves slowly so we have enough time at our disposal. Anxiety and the urgency of time leave us.

When we meditate we discover the infinite nature of our mind, and we become aware of the spiritual part of ourselves, which is our true nature.

THE HEALING POWER OF HUMOR

We always have choices. And one choice we have is to be happy independently from people and circumstances. We can fill our minds with cheerful thoughts and we can develop a healthy sense of humor. Cardiac patients especially need to overcome "chronic seriousness," replacing it with joyful anticipation and occasions of laughter and good humor. A Chinese proverb proclaims, "Life itself cannot give you joy unless you really will it. Life just gives you time and space. It is up to you to fill it."

Here's how Doctors Berk and Tan of Loma Linda University describe the beneficial effects of laughing. Laughter:

- lowers your blood pressure
- boosts your immune system
- decreases stress hormone production
- unleashes the flow of beta endorphins, the body's chemicals that leave us feeling euphoric.

In the Bible we read: "A merry heart is good medicine." Joy has been identified as a sign of God's presence. And it has been said that angels can fly because they take themselves lightly.

We also find humor in the words of patients: "The nurse gave me nine tablets I had to take altogether. They were a meal in itself." A five-year-old child told her grandma: "Next time, come and see my doctor. You won't have to wait and he will give you a lollypop."

And here's a a humorous story told by an airline pilot. It's based on a dream he had when he was admitted to the CCU. He calls it "Life at the Take Fun Away Hospital" and it's one of my personal favorites. I hope it makes you smile.

GOOD MORNING, FOLKS. This is your captain speaking. Welcome to the Cardiac Care Unit at Take Fun Away Hospital. This is Deadly Scare, your head nurse speaking. The CCU stay is like a voyage into the unknown, so I ask you to direct your attention to the nurse attendant for further instructions.

You will be staying at an altitude of three and a half feet, the temperature is 65 degrees, and there will be no wind. This is a nonsmoking CCU—it is strictly forbidden to smoke in the lavatory. Although smoking is prohibited, smoke alarms may go off.

There is only one exit, the front door, so please do not leave your bed until notified to do so. Your pillow can be used as a flotation device if the faucet overflows. On your right you have a beautiful view of the parking lot and on your left a pink wall.

Stow all luggage under your bed or in the compartment above your head. Visiting hours are from 3:30 P.M. to 4:30 P.M.

The CCU is fully equipped with credit card telephones. If you have chest pain, dial one. If you have shortness of breath, dial two, and then secure the mask located in the yellow bag above your head to your mouth for oxygen delivery. If you have any small children who need assistance, leave them at home.

Daily weigh-ins will take place at 5:00 A.M. sharp and breakfast will be served at 7:00 A.M.

Blood samples will be drawn throughout the day and night. Please be sure to get plenty of rest. If you are a frequent CCU attendee, notify the head nurse at once. We realize the CCU stay is expensive and ask you to save all urine. Your stay in the CCU will be about two weeks. Fifteen minutes prior to leaving you will be given further instructions.

We thank you again for staying at the Take Fun Away Hospital CCU. We know that you have a choice among hospital CCUs and we appreciate that you chose Take Fun Away Hospital. If we can be of further assistance, please do not hesitate to call on us. The head nurse and hospital crew wish you a pleasant day.

Nurse attendant, prepare for laundry.

YOUR HEART GIFT

This exercise is designed simply to bring to mind a moment in your life when you felt touched to the core of your being, when you were most yourself, perhaps expressing a natural talent, and to recognize what made it so meaningful.

Exercise

Seek in your spiritual heart the greatest gift you have received from God. Remember the circumstances of the occasion, who you were with, perhaps, or what you were doing. And then simply acknowledge it with gratitude.

MINDFULNESS

Our mind naturally wanders. Most of the time, it seems, our attention is uncontrolled. The mind is like a boat moved about by changing winds. We can awaken our consciousness and master our attentiveness with the practice of mindfulness.

Meditation

Don't miss your appointment with life—
practice mindfulness.
To be mindful means to live fully
in the present moment.
Most of the time,
our minds are focused on hardships of the past
or troubles of the future.
We are here, but not exactly here—
our mind wanders.

We are with our children,
*   but we miss their beautiful smile.*
They glue their eyes to our face in search of love.
They hug us to hold us in the present,
*   but we shake ourselves off*
*   to continue our rhythm of life.*
We miss the present moment,
*   the most important moment,*
*   the only certain moment.*
As we immerse ourselves in this reality
*   we capture life, as it is,*
*   in its full potential*
*   with its boundless creativity.*
Fill your life with these moments,
*   feel the present;*
You will live life fully.
Life will be long and without regrets.

CHAPTER NINE

Daily Spirituality

"When you search for me, you will find me;
if you seek me with all your heart."
—Jeremiah 29:13

Daily Habits

For a period of time, I had the experience of waking up in the morning with thoughts assaulting me. Worries about the hospital, patients, and publications—worries and more worries. I finally realized one day that this way of thinking was damaging.

Eventually, I developed the habit of starting the morning with positive thoughts: thanking God for another day of life and all the graces I received. I began reading material that was spiritually nourishing and uplifting. In addition, I started to meditate and listen to the quiet voice within. There is a reference in the Bible that says: "I am with you always, even up to the end of the world" (Matthew 28:20).

My meditation in the morning is a time of atonement. I remind myself that I am part of the Spirit of God. I sense his presence. I perceive his divine guidance. I find peace. To me, this practice is the most nourishing time of my day.

DAILY STEPS

We all believe that there is a God who is infinite love. Daily communion with this power gives us the faith to handle problems. It also helps to view problems as opportunities. We can ask ourselves, "What can I learn from this situation? How can I turn things around so that this experience will be a positive one for me?"

Another way to face uncertainty is to focus on our goals. When we have goals, we have a destination and all the other elements that can interfere become less powerful. If my destination is clear I lose sight of obstacles. One of the most helpful tools we have is to believe in God who is omnipresent, omnipotent.

A few days ago, in the hospital, I saw a patient on oxygen. He had lung cancer and it had spread to the brain, leaving him unable to move. He was reduced to lying in bed all the time, but his blue eyes showed a peaceful expression. I asked him how he felt inside. He looked straight at me and said without hesitation, "I feel wonderful. I leave everything in the hands of God." I was captured by the sense of peace and tranquility I saw in his eyes and the faith I heard in his words.

THE SEASONS OF THE HEART

A good way to focus on our goals is as if we were preparing for another season of rest and growth, another season where the

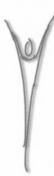

You can let worries consume you, or you can be attentive to your spiritual heart. You will experience ups and downs, seasons of the heart, seasons of winter and harshness, seasons of spring and new life. Your spiritual heart is the guardian of your physical well-being, so as you raise your level of consciousness, you can free yourself and change your life circumstances.

spirit enfolds within itself new manifestations, new expressions, new states of being. These are the seasons of our heart. They repeat themselves constantly, automatically. We cannot resist them, like we cannot resist the crashing waves of the ocean. So it is easy for us to follow the motion and go with it. The language of the heart changes according to the seasons. Our body and our mind evolve according to the seasons with a harmony and a purpose that are beyond our understanding.

Why is this winter so long? we ask ourselves. When is spring coming? And then we look for summer. When the summer is too hot, fall is our salvation. Paradoxically, we always seem unsatisfied. But nature smiles at our impatience. It is as if the universe is telling us, "What needs to happen for you to understand the message, to raise your level of consciousness? How can you realize that you are all here for a purpose: to serve God and humanity, so that when all the seasons end you will be happy because your life has meaning?" We played a good role. In the role we chose, we made the world a better place and in the process we rose to higher levels of spirituality and love, that wonderful force that holds the universe together.

DAILY TRANQUILITY

If I ask the question, "What is it that I want from life?" the answer most likely would be to find peace. Implicit with this request is the idea that we are looking for something outside ourselves. For instance, we say, "How can I be peaceful with so many financial difficulties, if the children are worrisome? How can I be peaceful if my health is not perfect? and so on. We forget to discover the fundamental principle that peace is a state of mind already within us, if only we become aware and attune ourselves to it. We find serenity when, during meditation and prayer, we center ourselves and look at ourselves and others from the highest point of view, from our spiritual heart. It is then that we are able to hear with our mind's ear and see with our mind's eye. As we raise our level of consciousness, we reach a higher degree of spiritual acceptance of ourselves. And in the silence of our heart we find peace.

YOUR HEART AS GUARDIAN

Here is a list of questions to help you see how the spiritual heart is the guardian of your physical heart. Take some time with these questions. Come back to them from time to time.

Exercise

1. *What do you do to physically protect your heart? (i.e. not smoking, watching cholesterol intake, maintaining weight, avoiding stress, social isolation, or hostility).*

2. *Is your daily life in line with your spiritual values?*
3. *Are you expressing these values and fulfilling them?*
4. *Are you giving yourself the love you need?*
5. *Are there any blocks to this love?*
6. *What about your love for others? Are you holding this love back?*
7. *What is most important for you to accomplish before you die?*
8. *What are you waiting for?*

As I write these questions, I have just finished working the garden in my back yard. I wonder, aren't our hearts in need of the same spiritual nourishment as our gardens? Don't our spiritual hearts also need to be watered and fed?

Imagine your spiritual heart as a tree. When you look down a street, you see trees in all shapes and sizes: some are large, some small; some extend themselves fully, reaching to a high point; others are smaller, dwarfed trees. Has your heart's spiritual growth been stunted? Or is it growing unbounded?

Bottom line: All of our lives are grounded in our relationship with God and this relationship lies in the spiritual heart.

THE WORLD OF ILLUSION

The Dalai Lama once said that the purpose of life is to seek happiness. Happy people are naturally friendly, creative, and

145

sensitive to others' needs. The highest happiness is to be free from bondage, to be liberated. True happiness is linked to the heart and mind more than the material world. Only in the spiritual domain does happiness remain unaffected by changing life circumstances.

Meditation

In spite of all the differences among human beings,
  we share fundamental needs:
  the need for peace,
  the need for love,
  and the need for happiness.
When I think about how much of my life I spend
  trying to satisfy these desires,
  tears run down my face.
How many steps I have taken.
How many words I have uttered.
Only to realize that in the world of control and power
  there is never an end;
  it is a world of illusion.
The true reality is the spiritual life.
In the spiritual domain
  we know ourselves
  and what God wants from us.
We realize that we have arrived,
  that we are at home
  and finally at peace,
  embraced by God's eternal love.

CHAPTER TEN

Conversations with God

"I asked my heart, 'How are you?'
'Expanding,' he answered,
'for I am the home of God.' "
—RUMI

DO WE NEED TO TALK TO GOD?

The answer is a resounding Yes!

And where do we encounter God? We meet God in our spiritual heart. The spark of life is in our heart and no one controls our heart but God. When we go beyond the ego and search in our heart, it is there that we encounter the divine.

The heart is the ground where the seed of our spirituality blooms. We all long for a union with the infinite, but this experience is a path that each of us must choose to follow. We achieve this spiritual connection when we embrace the silence and look into our heart for direction and guidance.

When we enter into meditation, in that silence within our heart, we can hear the voice of God. In the silence we can worship God. As a corollary to this experience, we discover our true self. This is where our spirituality sparkles. In this center lies our uniqueness. We have been created in God's own image.

PREPARING TO PRAY

Prayer is a movement in consciousness. Prayer is love in search of words. In the depths of our heart we seek communion with the divine in faith and trust, letting God become our soul companion. Through prayer we accept our spiritual nature and our purpose in life. We express our true self with God-centered consciousness. We pray also when we see the beauty of nature: the trees, the sky, the infinity of the sea, or the majesty of the mountains.

There is no specific time for prayer. We can close our eyes and immediately get in touch with the spirit within us. Express a thought and this is a prayer. We pray silently in meditation.

I am reminded of Janet, a forty-three-year-old woman who underwent mitral valve replacement at the age of twenty-two and again ten years later when she developed congestive heart failure. Her condition then significantly improved: she was happy, smiling, and symptom free. She opened her heart to me and said: "I take one day at a time. I pray incessantly. I ask God to give me the strength to sustain my life. When I experience a burst of energy, I praise the Lord."

I also recall Doctor Ralph J. Byrd, a San Francisco physician who studied three hundred ninety-three patients who were admitted to the hospital for heart attacks. He divided them into two groups. One group sought traditional medicine. The other group, in addition to medical attention, received prayers from an outside group unknown to them. The study showed that there was a statistically significant difference. The ones who received intercessory prayer left the hospital sooner.

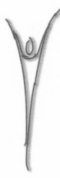

*Y*ou need to talk to God and you will discover his presence in your spiritual heart. But if you found yourself in the presence of God, what would you say? What would you do? Ask your spiritual heart. There is no time when you cannot communicate with God and seek communion with God through prayer. God is as close to you as your breath, silently waiting to be discovered.

They had fewer incidences of respiratory problems or cardiac problems. It was like a miracle.

Look at Yourself in the Mirror

Our mind, driven by the ego, is by nature judgmental and never fully satisfied. As we look at our reflection in a mirror, our tendency is to focus on our physical imperfections, and we feel the need to correct them. In the following exercise you are invited to see beyond the body and embrace your spiritual dimension.

Exercise

Each time you look in the mirror, think of yourself as seeing the Spirit of God within you. Don't let your gaze be distracted by your physical appearance. Don't judge yourself. Smile and hug yourself. Love is what we need the most.

Intimacy with God

As I woke up this morning a thought came into my mind: If I had to be in the presence of God, what would I say? As I was meditating on this, I realized that I was in the presence of God at that moment. I am in the presence of God at this moment. We all are in the presence of God at every instant of our lives, whether we are aware of it or not. I realized then that God gives us all our lives, an opportunity to be aware of him, his infinite love, his presence.

I have a vivid memory of an experience that happened only once in my life. I was at Hilton Head, South Carolina, in a hotel room. All of a sudden during my meditation, I experienced a state of higher consciousness. I became infinitely happy, profoundly peaceful. I felt a degree of joy that had no equal in my memories of the past. Never had I experienced such jubilation or deeper peace.

I remember distinctly that I had no desires, none. That state of mind was so fulfilling that there was nothing left to desire. I felt no more need to be successful, to be happy, to realize my dreams. They were all completed. This state of mind overshadowed all my needs and desires. It was a moment in which, for the first time in my life, I felt I could completely accept myself. There were no areas in my personality, or my body, nothing about myself, that needed to be changed. Everything seemed completely satisfactory.

Then I felt an intense love and unity with the universe. It included everyone. It was a stage which was beyond forgiveness. I had nothing to forgive. That state of consciousness was higher than forgiveness. It was a state of bliss, a state of universal consciousness. Never have I felt closer to God, and I thanked God in tears for having given me the privilege of experiencing such a state, something that transcends human experience. It was divine, but it was now my very own encounter.

While my eyes were still closed, I grabbed my tape recorder and described my feelings, hoping that I would be able to recall at will those very moments with the same wonderful beauty. I said to myself that if God, at this instant, would take me away, it would have been during the most enjoyable moment of my life. So pure. So totally fulfilling. So uncontaminated by the daily reality.

If I ask myself now to explain the whole experience, I can briefly summarize it in this simple phrase: "a change of consciousness." It was a change in awareness. I have never felt that I was more present in my heart than at that moment. I was totally in my heart. My heart was the center of love. That immense love had the infinite power of propelling me like an object, high in consciousness, to enjoy heights, feelings, and a pure state of being that were unknown to me before.

Later, I went down to the beach and rented a bike. With the joy of a child I began riding and as I was encountering people they looked different to me. Different in that I felt very close to each person I met. Everybody was smiling at me, as I was smiling at them. I saw couples. People of all ages were walking along the beach on that beautiful day, enjoying nature. I rode the bike for a long distance until the place where I had started from became so small behind me that I had to turn back.

In turning around, as I looked toward the ocean, I saw two dolphins swimming together. From time to time they would come out of the water and they seemed to hang suspended in the air. Then they would dive again. They looked so happy to me. Everything around me was filled with cheerfulness, harmony, peace, and love.

Gradually, this blissful state of mind lessened, but the memory of it has never left me. I recognized what was possible. I discovered the joy that my spiritual heart could offer me. A happiness without judgment. A blissfulness that had no time or space, a delight of infinite magnitude. All I remember now is the source. And the source is my spiritual heart.

I ask myself, why me? All I can say is that it happened. I know now that when you are in the presence of God you are alone. You are alone with God. It is like being on top of the highest mountain in the universe and you contemplate all around you, and that is all that you can see. I am grateful, O Lord, for this gift of love.

The fact that I had this experience means that God reveals himself to anyone who seeks him. As you seek God, God will answer you. God is as close to us as our breath. He is always there, silent, waiting to be discovered.

SELF-KNOWLEDGE THROUGH PRAYER

One of the most gratifying experiences is to seek God's wisdom and guidance, and then to sense his presence. Thank God for the miracle of life and express your deepest gratitude for his constant help.

Meditation

The key to prayer is to find a quiet place
where you can meditate.
When I ponder about the angel of God,
I experience a sense of complete peace.

My mind and my body are filled with love.
I am conscious that these spiritual elements
    are within me.
I do not pray to obtain things
    or to alter circumstances.
I pray to experience love and serenity.

O God, in the comfort of your peace
    all becomes clear and simple.
You satisfy that fundamental thirst
    to commune with your Spirit.
I close my eyes
    and my heart becomes suspended in air.
This freedom bathes me in joy and happiness.
It seems more real than the world;
    it's a reality within myself.
It's what we gain
    when we transcend our worldly needs
    and connect with our spiritual heart.

I realize that I can come back
    to this state of mind.
This can be part of my life.
In our divine heart we encounter God.
His immense and tender love
    fills our spiritual heart
    where healing happens.

Conclusion

FROM THE HEART

I felt compelled to write *The Spiritual Heart* for three reasons. First, I have been deeply affected by people dying of heart attacks or becoming invalids. I have come to realize that, in addition to medical care, people need an inner force that can assist them in recovery or in prevention of heart disease. This power is the spiritual heart. And this divine element brings an element of balance. It is the focus of our spiritual universe. Throughout our life we all need a spiritual refuge where we can find comfort and inspiration.

The second reason is that we need inner peace, the quality that we find in the spiritual heart. Inner peace comes with living in harmony with what we are meant to do in life—to serve God.

And finally, in this sacred domain we can hear the voice of God and become aware of his immense love. There will be a day, I believe, when the homage and respect for this power will become more accepted and an integral part of the practice of medicine.

If my words have been able to touch your heart, bring inner peace, and draw you closer to your spiritual heart, my mission is accomplished, and I thank you.

Recommended Reading

Benson, Dr. Herbert. *The Relaxation Response*, New York: Avon Book, 1976.
The learning and practice of a relaxation technique to cope with stress effectively.

Borysenko, Dr. Joan. *Guilt Is the Teacher, Love Is the Lesson*, New York: Warner Books, 1991.
A pathway to spiritual heights of self-acceptance and love.

Bovenmars, G., M.S.C. *A Biblical Spirituality of the Heart*, New York: Alba House, 1991.
This book illustrates the values and meaning of the heart in sacred scripture.

Chopra, Deepak. *Healing the Heart: A Spiritual Approach to Reversing Coronary Disease*, New York: Harmony Books, 1998.
A psychological and spiritual guide to preventing and healing heart disease based on the principles of ayurvedic medicine, meditation and self-awareness.

_____, *How to Know God: The Soul's Journey into the Mystery of Mysteries*, New York: Harmony Books, 2000.
A scientific approach to how we can know God and how we can experience God.

Cortis, Dr. Bruno. *Heart & Soul: A Psychological and Spiritual Guide to Preventing and Healing Heart Disease*, New York: Villard Books, 1995.

Cortis, Dr. Pia. *The Uncut Rose: Pathway to the Unhindered Expression of Feelings.*
Unpublished manuscript.

Dossey, Dr. Larry. *Healing Words: The Power of Prayer and the Practice of Medicine*, Harper SanFrancisco, 1993.
The scientific and spiritual approach to the power of prayer.

Frank, Arthur. *At the Will of the Body: Reflections on Illness*, New York: Houghton Mifflin, 1991.
This title explores the needs of a person who suddenly becomes a patient.

Gibran, Kahlil. *The Treasured Writings of Kahlil Gibran*, Secaucus, NJ: Castle Books, 1995.
Inspiring poems containing Eastern wisdom.

Hann, Thich Nhat. *The Present Moment: A Retreat on the Practice of Mindfulness*, Audio Book, Sounds True Recording, 1994.
The present is the only moment there is.

Hildebrand, Dietrich Von. *The Sacred Heart: Source of Christian Affectivity*, Baltimore, MD–Dublin, Ireland: 1965.
A treatise on the transforming power of Christ's love.

Jampolsky, Dr. Gerald. *Love Is Letting Go of Fear*, Berkeley, CA: Celestial Hearts, 1979.
Twelve lessons for personal transformation and inner peace.

Kornfield, Jack. *After the Ecstasy, the Laundry: How the Heart Grows Wise on the Spiritual Path*, New York: Bantam Books, 2000.
A pathway to wellness through personal development and inner transformation while facing the imperfection of daily life.

Legato, Marianne J., M.D., and Colman, Carol. *The Female Heart: The Truth about Women and Coronary Heart Disease*, New York: Simon and Schuster, 1991.
This book illustrates how women are susceptible to heart disease and how high-risk women can survive.

Lesser, Elizabeth. *The New American Spirituality: A Seeker's Guide*, New York: Random House, 1999.
How to have a spiritual relationship with God, and how to create spiritual freedom.

Mercer, Dr. Michael and Troiani, Dr. Maryann. *Spontaneous Optimism: Proven Strategies for Health, Prosperity and Happiness*, Castlegate Publishers, Inc., 1998.
A pathway to happiness and prosperity. Shows you how to create your own life.

Missildine, W. Hugh. *Your Inner Child of the Past*, New York: Simon and Schuster, 1963.
How to recognize and accept your inner child of the past.

Ornish, Dean, M.D. *Love and Survival: The Scientific Basis of the Healing Power of Intimacy*, New York: Harper Collins, 1998.
Intimacy, relationship, and love can heal our spiritual hunger and isolation.

Paddison, Sara. *The Hidden Power of the Heart: Achieving Balance and Fulfillment in a Stressful World*, Boulder Creek, CA: Planetary Publications, 1995.
How your heart wisdom can transform your life.

Rinpoche, Sogyal. *The Tibetan Book of Living and Dying*, HarperSanFrancisco, 1998.
How to understand the meaning of life, help the dying, and accept death.

158

Siegel, Dr. Bernie S. *Peace, Love and Healing*, New York: Harper and Row, 1989.
Illustrates the path to self-healing with profound humanity and practical wisdom.

Sylvia, Claire, with Novak, William; foreword by Bernie S. Siegel. *A Change of Heart: A Memoir*, New York: Little, Brown and Company, 1997.
The author opens our spirit to the possibility that cellular memory can outlive physical death.

Teasdale, Wayne. *The Mystic Heart: Discovering a Universal Spirituality in the World's Religions*, Novato, CA: New World Library, 1999.
This book addresses the transforming power of the Divine in human life and illustrates how the spiritual traditions are connected.

Whitehead, Carleton. *Creative Meditation*, New York: Dodd, Mead. 1975.
Learn how to attune yourself to the universal power and gain control of your life through creative meditation.

Zukav, Gary and Frances, Linda. *The Heart of the Soul: Emotional Awareness*, New York: Simon and Schuster, 2001.
How to align your personality with your soul.

Zukav, Dr. Gary. *The Seat of the Soul*, New York: Simon and Schuster, 1989.
The road to wisdom is through the heart.

Healing the Heart Seminar

This workshop speaks to our deepest needs for meaning, forgiveness, and love. It teaches how to know your heart, how to take care of it, and that the healing of the physical heart lies in the healing of your spiritual heart. The principles you learn will add years to your life and joy to your heart.

The Exceptional Heart Patients Program

This program gives hope and directions toward wellness by teaching you to be responsible for your health and to discover the ability to use your own healing power.

Invitation to Contact the Author:

Readers interested in knowing more about these programs, or who wish to share their own experiences in healing, are invited to write the author at:

Dr. Bruno Cortis
7605-1/2 West North Avenue
River Forest, Illinois 60305

You may access his website at:
http://www.imindhealth.com

Or send an e-mail to:
MindHealth@aol.com